first place
4 health

Bible Study Series

God's best for

your life

Janet Thompson

Published by Gospel Light
Ventura, California, U.S.A.
www.gospellight.com
Printed in the U.S.A.

Caution: The information contained in this book is intended to be solely for
informational and educational purposes. It is assumed that the First Place 4 Health
participant will consult a medical or health professional before beginning this or
any other weight-loss or physical fitness program.

Library of Congress Cataloging-in-Publication Data
Thompson, Janet.
God's best for your life.
p. cm. — (First place 4 health Bible study series)
ISBN 978-0-8307-5641-4
1. Christian women—Religious life—Textbooks. 2. Christian women—Health and
hygiene—Textbooks. 3. Christian life—Biblical teaching—Textbooks. I. Title.
BV4527.T475 2010
248.8'43—dc22
2010032982

Rights for publishing this book outside the U.S.A. or in non-English
languages are administered by Gospel Light Worldwide, an international
not-for-profit ministry. For additional information, please visit
www.glww.org, email info@glww.org, or write to Gospel Light Worldwide,
1957 Eastman Avenue, Ventura, CA 93003, U.S.A.

To order copies of this book and other Gospel Light products in bulk
quantities, please contact us at 1-800-446-7735.

contents

about the author

Janet Thompson, a graduate of Fuller Theological Seminary, is a popular conference speaker and author of 12 books, including the *Woman to Woman Mentoring: How to Start, Grow and Maintain a Mentoring Ministry* resources; *Dear God, They Say It's Cancer; Praying for Your Prodigal Daughter;* and several books in the New Hope Bible Studies for Woman series, *Face-to-Face*. She is also a contributing author in several other books. Janet, a wife, mother of four and grandmother of 11, writes and speaks from her home in Southern California. You can visit her ministry, About His Work Ministries, at www.womantowomanmentoring.com.

foreword

My introduction to Bible study came when I joined First Place in March 1981. I had been attending church since I was a small child, but the extent of my study of the Bible had been reading my Sunday School quarterly on Saturday night. On Sunday morning, I would listen to my Sunday School teacher as she taught God's Word to me. During the worship service, I would listen to our pastor as he taught God's Word to me. Frankly, the idea of digging out the truths of the Bible for myself had never entered my mind.

Perhaps you are right where I was back in 1981. If so, you are in for a blessing you never dreamed possible. As you start studying the truths of the Bible for yourself through the First Place 4 Health Bible studies, you will see God begin to open your understanding of His Word.

Almost every First Place 4 Health member I have talked with about the program says, "The weight loss is wonderful, but the most important thing I have received from my association with First Place 4 Health is learning to study God's Word." The First Place 4 Health Bible studies are designed to be done on a daily basis. As you work through each day's study (which will take 15 to 20 minutes to complete), you will be discovering the deep truths of God's Word. A part of each week's study will also include a Bible memory verse for the week.

There are many in-depth Bible studies on the market. The First Place 4 Health Bible studies are not designed for the purpose of in-depth study, but are designed to be used in conjunction with the rest of the program to bring balance into your life. Our desire is for each member to begin having a personal quiet time with God each day. This time alone with God should include a time of prayer, Bible reading and Bible study. Having a quiet time is a daily discipline that will bring the rich rewards of balance, which is something we all need.

God bless you as you begin this exciting journey toward a balanced life. God will richly bless your efforts to give Him first place in your life. Remember Matthew 6:33: "But seek first his kingdom and his righteousness, and all these things will be given to you as well."

Carole Lewis, First Place 4 Health National Director

introduction

First Place 4 Health is a Christ-centered health program that emphasizes balance in the physical, mental, emotional and spiritual areas of life. The First Place 4 Health program is meant to be a daily process. As we learn to keep Christ first in our lives, we will find that He is the One who satisfies our hunger and our every need.

This Bible study is designed to be used in conjunction with the First Place 4 Health program but can be beneficial for anyone interested in obtaining a balanced lifestyle. The Bible study has been created in a five-day format, with the last two days reserved for reflection on the material studied. Keep in mind that the ultimate goal of studying the Bible is not only for knowledge but also for application and a changed life. Don't feel anxious if you can't seem to find the *correct* answer. Many times, the Word will speak differently to different people, depending on where they are in their walk with God and the season of life they are experiencing. Be prepared to discuss with your fellow First Place 4 Health members what you learned that week through your study.

There are some additional components included with this study that will be helpful as you pursue the goal of giving Christ first place in every area of your life:

- **Group Prayer Request Form:** This form is at the end of each week's study. You can use this to record any special requests that might be given in class.

- **Leader Discussion Guide:** This discussion guide is provided to help the First Place 4 Health leader guide a group through this Bible study. It includes ideas for facilitating a First Place 4 Health class discussion for each week of the Bible study.

- **Two Weeks of Menu Plans with Recipes:** There are 14 days of meals, and all are interchangeable. Each day totals 1,400 to 1,500 calories and includes snacks. Instructions are given for those who need more calories. An accompanying grocery list includes items needed for each week of meals.

- **First Place 4 Health Member Survey:** Fill this out and bring it to your first meeting. This information will help your leader know your interests and talents.

- **Personal Weight and Measurement Record:** Use this form to keep a record of your weight loss. Record any loss or gain on the chart after the weigh-in at each week's meeting.

- **Weekly Prayer Partner Forms:** Fill out this form before class and place it into a basket during the class meeting. After class, you will draw out a prayer request form, and this will be your prayer partner for the week. Try to call or email the person sometime before the next class meeting to encourage that person.

- **Live It Trackers:** Your Live It Tracker is to be completed at home and turned in to your leader at your weekly First Place 4 Health meeting. The Tracker is designed to help you practice mindfulness and stay accountable with regard to your eating and exercise habits. Step-by-step instructions for how to use the Live It Tracker are provided in the *Member's Guide*.

- **Let's Count Our Miles!** A worthy goal we encourage is for you to complete 100 miles of exercise during your 12 weeks in First Place 4 Health. There are many activities listed on pages 255-256 that count toward your goal of 100 miles. When you complete a mile of activity, mark off the box listed on the Hundred Mile Club chart located on the inside of the back cover.

- **Scripture Memory Cards:** These cards have been designed so you can use them while exercising. It is suggested that you punch a hole in the upper left corner and place the cards on a ring. You may want to take the cards in the car or to work so you can practice each week's Scripture memory verse throughout the day.

- **Scripture Memory CD:** All 10 Scripture memory verses have been put to music at an exercise tempo in the CD at the back of this study. Use this CD when exercising or even when you are just driving in your car. The words of Scripture are often easier to memorize when accompanied by music.

welcome to
God's Best for Your Life

At your first group meeting for this session of First Place 4 Health, you will meet your fellow members, get an overview of your materials and find out what you can expect at weekly meetings. The majority of your class time will be spent learning about the four-sided person concept, the Live It Food Plan, and how change begins from the inside out. You will also have a chance to ask any questions about how to get the most out of First Place 4 Health. If possible, complete the Member Survey on page 205 before your first group meeting. The information that you give will help your leader tailor the next 12 weeks to the needs of the whole group.

Each weekly meeting begins with a weigh-in for members. This will allow you to track your progress over the 12-week session. Your Week One weigh-in/measurement will establish a baseline of comparison so that you can set healthy goals for this session. If you are apprehensive about weighing in every week, talk with your group leader about your concerns. He or she will have some options for you to consider that will make the weigh-in activity encouraging rather than stressful.

The day after your first meeting, begin Week Two of this Bible study. This session, you and your group will look at making healthy lifestyle choices to achieve God's best for your physical life. As you open yourself to the truth of Scripture and share your hopes and struggles with the members of your group during the next 12 weeks, you'll find yourself becoming the healthy child of God you are designed to be!

God's best for your physical life

SCRIPTURE MEMORY VERSE

Then Jesus declared, "I am the bread of life. He who comes to me will never go hungry, and he who believes in me will never be thirsty."

JOHN 6:35

I want to do what God wants me to do, but how do I know for sure what that is? I desire to live a life pleasing to God, but how will I know if I am pleasing Him? Does God want to be involved in every area of my life? What is God's plan for my life?

You have probably asked yourself some of these same questions, along with many others, while trying to figure out where to find the answers. If only you could ask God in person; if only there was a guidebook of instructions for living your life. Good news! God knows your questions, and His Word holds the answers. Your Bible provides everything you need to know about seeking God's best for *every* aspect of your life and for living a life that pleases and glorifies Him.

In order to learn God's best for your life, we'll delve into God's Word—specifically the book of Ruth—on a treasure hunt to discover the pearls of wisdom God has for each of us on the precious pages of our Bible and to discover the jewels of reward awaiting those who follow His directions. In preparation for this study, *God's Best for Your Life,* read Ruth (it's only four chapters long). Ruth exemplifies the fact that God rewards those who are obedient and conform their life to His will. A sincere desire to seek His will and accept what He reveals is the only requirement for discovering God's best for Your life.

YOUR BODY—GOD'S GIFT

Dear Lord, You have entrusted me with a unique physical body. Help me to treasure my body as much as You do and to treat it with respect. Amen.

One time an old Sunday School teacher told some of his Sunday School boys the biblical reference for next Sunday's lesson. As a prank, the boys stole his Bible and glued together several pages of next Sunday's text.

The following Sunday, the teacher started reading from his Bible. When he reached the bottom of the page he read, "When Noah was 120 years old he took unto himself a wife, who . . ." Turning the glued-together page, he continued, ". . . was 140 cubits long, forty cubits wide, built of gopher wood, and covered with pitch inside and out." The teacher paused, and with a puzzled expression, read it again. Then he said, "My friends, this is the first time I have ever seen this in the Bible, but I take it as evidence of the assertion that we are fearfully and wonderfully made!"

Those kids played a joke on their Sunday School teacher, who didn't seem to notice he was describing the ark instead of Noah's wife. Or maybe he knew he'd been tricked and seized the opportunity to make the point that no matter what our dimensions, God made us all.

When you joined your First Place 4 Health group, you took a giant step toward seeking God's best for your physical life. Read Psalm 139:13-16. What reasons do you have to praise God?

_____

_____

_____

_____

What about you is "fearfully and wonderfully made"?

_____

_____

_____

_____

You are God's workmanship, and your body is a gift from God. God created your body fearfully and wonderfully in your mother's womb. When a baby is born, friends and family often exclaim to the parents, "You do good work! You made a beautiful baby." But the parents didn't really make that beautiful baby: God made the baby through the parents, who had the joy of birthing God's precious creation—the same way He made you. In whose image was the first human made, and how did God create the first human (see Genesis 1:27; 2:7)?

_____

_____

_____

_____

Describe several items that you've created from scratch.

_____

_____

_____

_____

When we invest time, energy and love into making something, we're proud of our creation and want it cared for properly. How does God want you to care for His creation—you, which He made from scratch?

_____

_____

_____

_____

Read Deuteronomy 32:6. How do you think God feels when you don't cherish His gift of your body?

_____

_____

_____

_____

Read 1 Corinthians 6:19-20. Why are you to honor God with your body?

_____

_____

_____

_____

My Creator, forgive me for not always showing respect to Your creation—my body. With Your help, I will do better in the future. Thank You for not giving up on me. Amen.

Day 2

HEAVENLY BREAD

Lord, I want to lavish my body with healthy foods. I truly seek Your best in this area, and I know I cannot be successful until I surrender my will to Your will. Speak to me as only You can. Amen.

Yesterday we talked about how God created our bodies, and today we'll talk about how He provided food and water to fuel our bodies and keep them functioning properly. Unfortunately, we often attach more meaning and uses for food than God ever intended. When God created man, He created a garden of food to sustain humans (see Genesis 1:29).

What else was in the Garden, and, according to Genesis 2:16-17, what warning did God give Adam?

_____

_____

_____

_____

Why didn't Adam and Eve heed God's warning (see Genesis 3:1-6)?

_____

_____

_____

_____

What were the results of choosing what *they thought* was best instead of what *God said* was best (see Genesis 3:22-24)?

_____

_____

_____

_____

Why did Elimelech and Naomi move their family from Bethlehem ("the house of bread") to the grain-filled, but pagan, land of Moab (see Ruth 1:1-2)?

_____

_____

_____

_____

What transpired in Moab, and why did Naomi return to Bethlehem (see Ruth 1:3-6)?

_____

_____

_____

_____

Adam and Eve missed God's intended best because they doubted God's word and disobeyed by eating forbidden food. God promised the Israelites abundant food if they remained obedient; a famine (such as described in Ruth 1:1) meant that the people had disobeyed God (see Deuteronomy 11:13-17). In both cases, doubting God's word and disobeying resulted in great suffering, pain and loss. Are you dissatisfied with God's provision of healthy food? Why or why not?

_____

_____

_____

_____

God's original plan called for man never to die; but in Adam and Eve's desire to be godlike, they ate the forbidden fruit and changed God's plans forever. Sin entered the world and mankind would need a redeeming Savior. So God sent His Son, Jesus Christ, to die a terrible death on the cross for our sins and to offer us forgiveness and eternal life (see John 3:16). In John 6:35, this week's memory verse, Jesus declared He is "the bread of life," and believing in Him means never being hungry or thirsty again. In what ways is Jesus "the bread of life"?

_____

_____

_____

_____

If you haven't accepted Christ as your Savior, now is the time to consider doing so. If you know you've sinned and need forgiveness, and you're ready to ask Jesus to come into your heart as your personal Savior—the Bread of Life—pray the Salvation Prayer given below right now. If you're a Christian but haven't been walking with Jesus as you know you should, pray this prayer as a rededication of your life to Christ.

> *Dear Jesus, I know that I have made mistakes and sinned in my life, and I am sorry. Please forgive me and cleanse me of those sins. Jesus, I want You to come into my heart. I believe You are the Son of God, that You died on the cross to pay the price for my sins, and You rose again in three days to offer me eternal life. Jesus, I willingly surrender my heart, mind and soul to You. Lord, I give You my life—make me a new creation in You. Amen.*

Congratulations! You've started a relationship that will sustain you through good times and bad. Know that God will never abandon you and is eager to help you succeed in all aspects of your life: physically, mentally, emotionally and spiritually. As you continue with this Bible study, you'll receive guidance for how to grow and mature your faith while you also learn how to live a healthy lifestyle.

Abba, Father, Thank You for being a loving, compassionate and forgiving God. I want to continue to grow closer to You as I learn how to take better care of myself, Your wonderful work. Amen.

HEALTH WATCH

Lord, I want to be healthy, but I face so many temptations every day. Help me stay strong physically and emotionally. With You beside me, I can overcome the obstacles that come between the way I want to live and the way I am living.

Mark Twain once said, "The only way to keep your health is to eat what you don't want, drink what you don't like and do what you'd rather not." We nervously laugh at Twain's comment, because it hits home. Many of us look at doing healthy things as punishment, and we call those who follow a healthy regimen "health nuts." We want to be healthy, but we don't want to do healthy. We may arrive at this crossroads because we think a healthy lifestyle involves eliminating fun and enjoyment, but actually the opposite is true: An unhealthy lifestyle undermines our joy and demoralizes us. God wants us to be healthy in both a physical sense and a spiritual sense, because He knows that the two are intertwined: Our physical life always affects our spiritual life, and vice versa.

Think about your physical condition. Are you fit or out of shape? Are you strong and vigorous or weak and rundown? Are you somewhere in between? Have you consulted with your doctor about where you need to be and how to get there?

_____

_____

_____

_____

Think about your spiritual condition. Are you active in your faith, or do you just go through the motions? Do you look forward to spending time alone with God, or do you regard it as a chore? Have you asked God for help and consulted the Bible to see what God says?

_____

_____

_____

_____

Read in Daniel 1:1-17 the story of Daniel's captivity and his choosing to live a healthy lifestyle, even when tempted with rich food. Daniel based his food choices on knowing God's best for his physical life. The royal foods were tainted because a portion of those foods was offered to the pagan gods, and because the meat was from unclean animals (by Jewish standards). How did Daniel describe what the royal food and wine would do to his body (see verse 8)?

_____

_____

_____

_____

What test did Daniel suggest (see verses 12-13)?

_____

_____

_____

What was the result at the end of 10 days (see verses 15-16)? How did God reward Daniel and the other three young men (see verse 17)?

_____

_____

_____

_____

Good health isn't solely dependent on food choices. Sufficient sleep is also essential, and numerous medical studies prove that eight hours of sleep a night helps weight loss. God designed our bodies to rebuild and refuel during sleep. What benefit of sleep is described in each of the following verses?

Psalm 3:5

_____
_____
_____

Psalm 4:8

_____
_____
_____

Proverbs 3:24

_____
_____
_____

Many of us try to extend our day by shaving off hours of sleep. How many hours of sleep do you average nightly? If you are averaging less than 8 hours, list four lifestyle changes you could make to add a half hour's sleep.

1. _____
2. _____
3. _____
4. _____

How would following Solomon's advice in Proverbs 3:7-8 help you to maintain a healthier body?

_____
_____
_____

Dear Father, I pray that I may enjoy good health and that all will be well with me, even as my soul is getting well (see 3 John 1:2). Amen.

Day 4 BEING FIT FOR LIFE

Lord, I want to become physically fit. Guide me as I make exercise a priority in my life, and help me discover a physical activity that I enjoy. Amen.

People either enjoy exercise, work out to an obsessive extreme, exercise out of duty, or think it's an unnecessary waste of time. What do you think of exercise? Why?

_____

_____

_____

_____

With today's many technological advances, time-saving devices and transportation options, we have to work to keep our bodies fit and functioning properly. Use the chart below to document what you do during a typical day. After each activity, tell how many minutes you spent doing it and tell whether it was a sedentary activity or a physical activity.

Date: _____

Activity	Minutes spent	Sedentary or physical

Now total the number of minutes spent doing each type of activity:

Sedentary activities   =   _____ minutes

Physical activities   =   _____ minutes

Decide how many minutes you want to knock off the total time spent on sedentary activities and add to your physical activities total. Keep this goal in mind as you start seeking God's best for your life.

We don't read much about exercise in the Bible because during that time, daily life provided sufficient exercise. Imagine the upper body strength of Ruth from gleaning and carrying home almost 50 pounds of barley (see Ruth 2:17-18). When Naomi and Ruth moved from Moab to Bethlehem, their trip probably took them 7 to 10 days of steadily walking over rugged and steep terrain. So Naomi, an older woman, was probably as fit as Ruth.

Except for Palm Sunday's triumphant entry on a donkey, the Gospels describe Jesus walking. Here is a sampling of Scriptures illustrating Jesus walking while ministering:

As Jesus was _____ beside the Sea of Galilee, he saw two brothers, Simon called Peter and his brother Andrew (Matthew 4:18).

As he _____ along, he saw Levi son of Alphaeus sitting at the tax collector's booth. "Follow me," Jesus told him, and Levi got up and followed him (Mark 2:14).

Afterward Jesus appeared in a different form to two of them while they were _____ in the country (Mark 16:12).

Read the following Scriptures. What point is being made about walking?

Deuteronomy 5:33

_____

_____

_____

Micah 6:8

_____

_____

_____

John 8:12

_____

_____

_____

1 John 1:7

_____

_____

_____

Read Ecclesiastes 4:9-10. What are the advantages of doing something with at least one other person?

_____

_____

_____

_____

_____

Friends can help us get on track and keep on track physically and spiritually, plus a lot of people find that exercising with a companion or two is more enjoyable than exercising alone. Consider pairing up with someone in your First Place 4 Health group to achieve your goal of 100 miles during the 12 weeks of this study (see "Let's Count Our Miles" in the back of this book). You don't have to join a gym, own elaborate equipment or dread your workout. The point is to keep moving.

Precious Jesus, help me stay firm in my walk with You
both physically and spiritually. Amen.

HOME, SWEET HOME

Father, I want our home to be a place of sweet accord but not abounding in sweets. I take seriously the task and privilege of feeding and caring for my family, and I know with Your help, I can instill healthy habits in my home.

Read Proverbs 31:10-31. Women often joke about only being Proverbs 31 Wannabes, because this biblical woman can seem intimidating. But some of you (and this includes men) *do* get up before dawn to provide food for your family, and you probably don't have "servant girls" (verse 15), so you need to think smart when it comes to maintaining your family's health. If you're a family of one or a single parent, you make all the food and health decisions for your family. In households like the Proverbs 31 family where the husband leaves home management to his wife, the husband has confidence that she will seek God's best for the family. Why did Mr. Proverbs 31 have confidence in his wife (see verses 11-12, 25-27)?

_____

_____

_____

What was the woman's reward for taking good care of her family (see verses 28,31)?

_____

_____

_____

_____

What do you consider your reward for caring for your family (or yourself, if you live alone)?

_____

_____

In a group of women who were studying the book *Loving Your Husband*, the most controversial session was the one on preparing nutritious meals for their family. Many participants said they didn't have the time, energy or *desire* to worry about feeding their family properly. You're in First Place 4 Health because you *do* care. Do you think your family would join you in following what God says about taking care of your body? Why or why not?

_____

_____

_____

_____

_____

How could you suggest changing to a healthy lifestyle in such a way that your family would accept it and look forward to the change? Would discussing statistics help? Would using different terms ("I-love-you-foods" instead of "healthy foods") work? What are some other ideas?

_____

_____

_____

_____

_____

We all desire God's best for our family, and yet, like Elimelech and Naomi, sometimes our actions don't result in a permanent solution. Overseeing the family's healthy lifestyle provides an awesome opportunity and responsibility to incorporate the principles of your First Place 4 Health program, no matter who in your family typically does the majority of shopping, menu planning and cooking. For each category in the chart on the following page, list the healthy lifestyle principle(s) you're applying and ones you want to add. (An example is provided to get you started.)

Category	Principle you are applying	Principle you want to add
Grocery shopping	*Using a list*	
Menu planning		
Cooking		
Snacks		
Family exercise		

Lord, I love my family, and I want only the best for them—as You do. Help me make wise choices and learn how to prepare healthy meals they'll enjoy. Thank You for caring about the food we eat, and thank You for my family.

REFLECTION AND APPLICATION

Day
6

Lord, I want to treat my body as a temple fit for and worthy of the Holy Spirit, but I know the work starts in my heart. Keep in me the desire to apply what I have learned this week to honor You with my body. Amen.

Professional bodybuilders work on many of the things we've talked about—proper nutrition, staying healthy, daily workouts, adequate sleep—but their motives are often to win contests, break records or achieve an extreme physique. Your motives are spiritual. Your reason for bodybuilding is to honor God by maintaining a body pleasing to Him—He designed your body for His glory. Remember, all your efforts are in vain if you don't include God in the building.

Every aspect of this week's study might not apply to your situation. As you reflect on what you've studied, pray about where you need to start.

Often, conquering one area will help lead to the next area—it's a process. For example, once you start exercising, you might find the endorphins kick in and you have more energy without feeling as if you need to fill yourself with empty calories, and you'll sleep better. Or you'll discover that proper nutrition gives you more energy to exercise. You get the idea. God wants you to be successful, but you must include Him in the process.

After each of the following verses, write a prayer asking God, the Master Builder of everything, to be a part of your bodybuilding.

Psalm 127:1

_____
_____
_____

Luke 6:46-49

_____
_____
_____

Hebrews 3:4

_____
_____
_____

God, my Creator, motivate me, guide me, sustain me, rebuild me. Amen.

Day 7 REFLECTION AND APPLICATION

Lord, You assure me that You are ready to answer my questions and guide me in the ways best for my body, for my life and for the lives I influence. Amen.

One of the biggest problems most people have when it comes to changing to and maintaining a healthy lifestyle is resisting temptation. Maybe you know you should exercise, but you figure that you'll take just today off and exercise twice as much tomorrow. Or rather than throwing out (or giving away) unhealthy food that is in your cupboard, you decide that you'll eat it instead. Or you're in a hurry and decide that "just this once" you'll have a donut (or two) for breakfast.

Temptation itself isn't the problem. Even Jesus was tempted. He spent 40 days and 40 nights in the desert and then was tempted by Satan three times—and the first temptation had to do with food! Each time, though, Jesus resisted and quoted Scripture. That's one of the reasons why memorizing Scripture is an important thing for you to do. Whenever you are tempted—whether it's to forego exercise or eat something you shouldn't—you can recall a Scripture verse, and God will help you overcome the temptation.

Read 1 Corinthians 10:13. What does this verse tell you about temptation and what God will do about it?

_____

_____

_____

_____

Jesus knows all about temptation, and He'll never let you be tempted beyond what you can resist. Remember, temptation is not a sin. The sin happens when you yield to temptation. Turn to Psalm 104:24-28. How does God care for everything He created?

_____

_____

_____

_____

Dear God, thank You for creating me just the way that You did. Thank You for always being there for me. Thank You for abundantly providing for all your creatures and for offering us eternal life. Thank You for loving me. I love You, too. Amen.

Group Prayer Requests

4 first place
health

Today's Date: _____

Name	Request

Results

_____
_____
_____
_____
_____
_____

God's best for your spiritual life

Scripture Memory Verse

"Ever since the time of your forefathers you have turned away from my decrees and have not kept them. Return to me, and I will return to you," says the Lord Almighty.

Malachi 3:7

We studied last week how God created us in His image, and this week we'll study how He created us to have a relationship with Him. But Satan also vies for a relationship with us, so we have a choice: a relationship with God or Satan? Good or evil? We have to choose one or the other—we can't hold hands with both.

In the Old Testament, God's people vacillated numerous times between relying on God and resenting God. When Naomi and her husband moved to a pagan land instead of remaining in God's Promised Land, their two sons married Moabite women and "turned away from my [God's] decrees" (see Deuteronomy 23:3-6; Malachi 2:11-12). Our memory verse this week, Malachi 3:7, is from the last of many Old Testament prophets God commissioned to forewarn His people about the consequences of their sin, but still they refused to listen. They hardened their hearts toward their Creator and paid the price: God went silent for 400 years!

God didn't speak again until He proclaimed through the angel Gabriel and the prophet John the Baptist that He was sending the Redeemer, Jesus Christ. Last week some of you accepted Jesus into your heart for the first time, and some of you rededicated your life to the Lord—praise God! For believers new and old alike, our memory verse will serve as a reminder that if you stray from obeying God's command-ments, you can return to Him, and He *will* return to you. He's been wait-ing for this moment. God only wants what's best for us, and to that end, He asks that we stay in relationship with Him. But how do we do that? That's what we will be learning this week—how to develop God's best for your spiritual life through a relationship with God, His Son (Jesus Christ) and the Holy Spirit.

If you're a new believer, this week will present you with guidelines for establishing and maintaining a relationship with God. If you're a sea-soned believer, this week will offer a renewed depth and freshness to your walk with the Lord. All God has ever wanted from His people is for us to honor, respect, trust and love Him above all earthly things, the same way He loves us. Everything—physical, emotional, relational, spiritual—stems from our devotion to Him. Nothing in our life will be right until we get it right with the Lord.

Day
1

CHANGING FROM THE INSIDE OUT

Lord, I'm aware of my tangible physical life, but often I forget that Your Spirit lives within me. Help me seek Your best for my spiritual life. Amen.

Our spiritual life is as visible as our physical life—it shows from the in-side out. Look up Ruth 1:16-18. How were Ruth's words and actions a statement of an inner faith?

_____

_____

_____

_____

_____

We learned last week that our body is a temple of the Holy Spirit. But where does the Spirit come from, and when do we get it? Read Acts 2:38 and then delineate the steps to take in order to become a Christian:

Step 1   _____ and be

Step 2   _____, every one of you, in the name of Jesus Christ
                for the forgiveness of your sins.

Step 3   And you will receive the gift of the _____ _____.

Repentance involves admitting our sins and asking for forgiveness. Baptism is an outward demonstration of an inward decision for Christ; it shows that we have repented and been forgiven. This then makes us clean and worthy of being a dwelling place for the Holy Spirit, which is a gift from God. What is the role of the Holy Spirit (see John 14:16-20,26)?

_____

_____

_____

_____

What kind of a relationship does Jesus want to have with His followers (see John 14:15,21,23)?

_____

_____

_____

_____

Read Galatians 5:19-21. What are the "obvious" signs of a person who is lacking a spiritual life and a relationship with Jesus?

_____

_____

_____

_____

Faith in Jesus Christ is visible. Turn to Galatians 5:22-23. In the first column, list the obvious signs of a spiritual life—the fruit of the Spirit—and in the second column, indicate work you need to do for the Holy Spirit to shine from your inside out.

The fruit of the Spirit	Work I need to do
1.	
2.	
3.	
4.	
5.	
6.	
7.	
8.	
9.	

According to Mark 7:14-20, how did Jesus use food to explain that the condition of our spiritual life is evident on the outside, that we can't hide our inner faith (or lack of it)?

_____

_____

_____

_____

What will be the result of practicing God's best for your spiritual life (see John 14:27)?

_____

_____

_____

_____

Holy Spirit, I want Your presence in my life to be visible from the inside out. Teach me, mold me and help me learn Your ways. Amen.

DRESSING FOR THE BATTLE

Lord, I want to grow in my spiritual life. My desire is to draw closer to You, but sometimes I feel as if You are distant and the world is near. Help me with this inner battle. I do love You, Lord. Amen.

Warren Wiersbe once said, "The Christian Life is not a playground; it is a battleground."[1] He was right, and most believers have recognized this for a long time. Just look at the titles found on some old hymns (like "Onward Christian Soldiers") and even in the name of some Christian organizations (like the Salvation Army). Some people believe the myth that Christians enjoy peace and tranquility and never have problems, but Jesus said, "In this world you will have trouble. But take heart! I have overcome the world" (John 16:33). When you gave your life to Christ, you also enlisted on the winning side in God's army!

According to 1 Peter 5:8, who do we fight?

> Be self-controlled and alert. Your enemy the _____ prowls around like a roaring lion looking for someone to devour.

Which fruit of the Spirit should we show? How hard is this to do when you're under attack?

_____

_____

_____

_____

Joshua 23:10 states that "the LORD your God fights for you, just as he promised," and He provides a battle plan in Ephesians 6:10-18, referred to as the "armor of God." Our spiritual armor mimics the defensive equipment worn by a Roman soldier during biblical times. Next to each piece of armor listed in the chart on the following page, indicate its spiritual application and its protection or purpose.

Piece of equipment	Spiritual application	Protection or purpose
Belt of Truth (v. 4)		
Breastplate of Righteousness (v. 14)		
Shoes of the Gospel of Peace (v. 15)		
Shield of Faith (v. 15)		
Helmet of Salvation (v. 17)		
Sword of the Spirit (v. 17)		

What does Paul remind us to do in Ephesians 6:18?

Pray in the _____ on _____ occasions with all kinds of _____
and _____. With this in mind, be _____ and _____ keep on
praying for all the _____.

Each day presents new battles, because Satan and his minions will never give up throwing temptation and other roadblocks your way. Write a short prayer that you can use to suit up spiritually every morning in the armor of God, alert and ready for whatever challenges come your way.

_____

_____

_____

_____

Satan doesn't want you to succeed in any spiritual endeavor, and certainly not in your First Place 4 Health program. How will knowing his strategy help you to confidently stand firm when facing life's choices and temptations?

_____

_____

_____

_____

Satan doesn't worry about those whose hearts have strayed, and he's not afraid of a dusty Bible. He targets spiritual warriors; but don't worry—Jesus has won the battle. Read Colossians 2:15. How did Jesus defeat Satan?

_____

_____

_____

Thank You, Lord, for being my protector, defender and shield. With Your Word in my heart, I can handle whatever life has in store for me. Amen.

CONFRONTING THE ENEMY

Day 3

Father, sometimes the enemy frightens me, and I don't know how to fight back. I don't want to give him that edge in my life. Teach me the tools of combat, and give me the insight and wisdom to use them. Amen.

You're suited up and standing firm in your spiritual armor. What is Satan's attack strategy? He'll send "flaming arrows"—temptations, troubles, threats and twisted truths—to hit where you're the weakest, most sensitive, and likely to turn away from the Lord's decrees, as God's people did in the time of Malachi. You may be thinking, *I would never do that!* That's exactly what Peter was probably thinking when he said to Jesus, "Even if all fall away, I will not" and "Even if I have to die with you, I will never disown you" (Mark 14:29,31). But when the going got tough, Peter surrendered to Satan. Fortunately, Peter learned from his failings and later taught the Early Church how to stand firm when facing the enemy.

Read Acts 4:1-20. How did Peter change?

_____

_____

_____

Peter matured in his faith by learning how to use the sword of the Spirit. Turn to Acts 2:14-41. How did Peter support what he had to say (see verses 16-21,25-31,34-36)?

_____

_____

_____

How did Peter quoting Old Testament Scriptures fulfill Isaiah 55:10-11?

_____

_____

_____

When Jesus was ready to start His ministry, the Holy Spirit led Him into the desert and allowed Satan to tempt Him (see Luke 4:1-13). What was the only offensive weapon Jesus used against Satan (see verses 4,8,12), and what was Satan's response (see verse 13)?

_____

_____

_____

The bad news is that Satan will be back at an "opportune time," but the good news is that we've got a Bible full of weapons to use against him. Why is memorizing Scripture so important and valuable (see Psalm 119:11)?

_____

_____

_____

How will memorizing this week's verse, Malachi 3:7, help you conquer a current temptation or help you make a right decision?

_____

_____

_____

_____

Pastor Charles Swindoll advises, "I know of no other single practice in the Christian life more rewarding, practically speaking, than memorizing Scripture."[2]

Father, help me hide Your Word in my heart, so when I'm tempted or don't know the right choice, Your wisdom fills my mind through the Scriptures I have memorized. Give me a burning desire to read my Bible. Amen.

FREEDOM THROUGH REPENTANCE — Day 4

Lord, I want to be successful in my First Place 4 Health program and in my walk with You. Please help me recognize acts of disobedience and experience the freedom of going beyond remorse to repentance. Amen.

J. Edwin Orr, a revivalist and historian, wrote the following about participating with Billy Graham in a revival attended by the notorious gangster Mickey Cohen:

He [Cohen] expressed some interest in the message, so several of us talked with him, including Dr. Graham, but he made no commitment until some time later when another friend urged him—with Revelation 3:20 as a warrant—to invite Jesus Christ into his life. This he professed to do, but his life subsequently gave no evidence of repentance, "the mighty change of mind, heart, and life." He rebuked our friend, telling him, "You did not tell me that I would have to give up my work!" He meant his rackets. "You did not tell me that I would have to give up my friends!" He meant his gangster associates. He had heard that so-and-so was a Christian cowboy, so-and-so was a Christian actress, so-and-so was a Christian senator, and he really thought he could be a Christian gangster.[3]

We may chuckle at the naivety of Mickey Cohen, but aren't we sometimes just as naïve? Do we abandon *all* habits or actions displeasing to God when we become Christians, or do we expect not to have to change in order to have a fruitful and meaningful spiritual life?

God's promise in this week's memory verse, "Return to me, and I will return to you," requires us to make the first move. God is waiting and watching. For new Christians and for Christians who have backslidden, old sinful ways must be replaced with new righteous ways. In Ruth 1:20-22, Naomi acknowledged that she was "full" before straying from the Lord's plan, but upon her return, she was humbled, repentant and "empty." (The Lord, however, did return to her in a mighty way.)

The Greek word for repentance is *metanoia,* which means "to think differently after"—a change of mind to turn from sin and do what's right. Look up "remorse" in a dictionary. What is the difference between "repentance" and "remorse"?

_____
_____
_____
_____

Look up "regret" in a dictionary. What is the difference between "repent" and "regret"?

_____
_____
_____
_____

Feeling sorry for something we've done simply leads to feelings of guilt, discouragement and depression and a probable repetition of the problem behavior. Describe a time when you experienced remorse or regret but didn't change and do what's right. What were the results?

_____

_____

_____

Our memory verse is from a time when the prophet Malachi addressed a people trying to make up for their sins by doing "right things"—going to the Temple and offering sacrifices—but their hearts were far from God and they had lost hope and faith in God and His promises. The Ephesians, who at one time had worshipped and served out of love for Jesus (see Ephesians 3:17-19) had a similar problem. Read Revelation 2:2-7. How did Jesus first commend the Ephesians (see verses 2-3)?

_____

_____

_____

For what did Jesus reprimand them (see verse 4)?

_____

_____

_____

According to verse 5, what two things were the Ephesians supposed to do?

_____

_____

_____

What warning and promise did they receive (see verse 7)?

_____

_____

_____

The key to the promise was *hearing* and *heeding* the warning. We may think that if we don't talk to God about our indiscretions, He won't know about them. Who is the only person we're fooling (see Jeremiah 23:23-24)?

_____

_____

_____

_____

Naomi knew she had displeased God and there were consequences, but she didn't stay away—she took the first step to return (see Ruth 1:20-22). Are you trying to hide anything from God? Have you eaten unhealthy food because you were alone and thought no one could see you? Did you really exercise for 30 minutes, or was it only for 10 minutes? Is there anything that is interfering with your relationship with God and with others? Spend some time today talking with God about any of these issues you find in your life.

> *Lord, I want to walk in the freedom that comes from reading, memorizing and following Your Word. Help me to be truly repentant and obedient. Amen.*

Day 5 — ENJOYING YOUR RELATIONSHIP WITH GOD

> *Lord, I want to find my joy in You and not in the world. Often I look to temporary earthly pleasures when You're ready to fill me with a never-ending joy that truly satisfies. Help me to choose wisely. Amen.*

God wants to share with us a relationship that is so fulfilling for us that we clap our hands and sing, "I have the joy, joy, joy, joy down in my heart to stay." The love of Jesus should radiate from our eyes and smile.

As you strive to achieve God's best for your life, your joy will increase proportionately. Doesn't that make you want to break out in song? It doesn't require a singing voice to make a joyful noise unto the Lord. Worshipping God in song and praise is one way of showing God how much you enjoy and love Him, and God rejoices with you.

King David was a poet and a harpist, and many of his psalms possess a theme of celebratory joy in following the Lord's commands. Read the Scriptures listed below and tell the reason why David experienced joy.

Scripture	Reason for joy
Ps. 5:11-12	
Ps. 16:11	
Ps. 19:8-11	
Ps. 28:6-7	
Ps. 95:1-3	

Look up Psalm 145:1-7 and Psalm 149:3. In what ways could you display joy in your relationship with God? Place a checkmark over each way that you have used. Circle a way you plan to try.

It's natural to focus on how the Lord makes *you* feel good, puts a smile on *your* face and keeps *you* happy. Have you given any thought to making God happy? Read Proverbs 10:1. What does a wise son bring to his father?

Because we are children of God, we should be wise and bring our heavenly Father the same thing. Our transgressions make Him sad, but when we repent and obey His commands, there's a party in heaven (see Luke

15:7). Read John 15:10. What must we do so that we remain in God's love and joy?

_____

_____

_____

Read Romans 14:17-18. What three things must we practice in order to please God?

_____

_____

_____

Read Nehemiah 8:10. What is our strength?

_____

_____

_____

What are the two greatest commandments (see Matthew 22:37-39)?

_____

_____

_____

> *Thank You, Lord, for wanting to share a joyful relationship with me. Help me to stay on Your paths and help me to show people how loving You are. I am so very grateful that You're my Father and that You saved me. Amen.*

Day 6 — REFLECTION AND APPLICATION

Abba, Father, Savior, Redeemer. I want to savor You more than what the world has to offer. You deserve all the honor, glory and praise. Amen.

God's best for your life is all about relationship—with others and with God. When we accept Jesus as our Savior, we become His children. This establishes the relationship, but, like all children, we don't always do the right thing. Maybe we don't exercise as much as we should. Maybe we fudge a little on the portions of food we eat. Maybe we think, *I don't see anyone I know around me, so I'll have that rich dessert that I crave.*

God knows that we're not perfect, but He does want us to own up to those times when we slip. We need to confess our sins, change our ways and prepare for the ensuing spiritual battle that could cause us to fall again and require repentance. God loves us so much—in fact, so much so that He has given us spiritual armor to help us ward off the temptations and lies that Satan flings at us. All we need to do is return to God—and He will return to us.

This week, we've also learned that our spiritual relationship with God is full of joy. We bring God joy when we obey His commands and show love to each other. God's joy, in turn, gives us strength.

Today, spend time alone with God singing praise songs and thanking Him for the many wonderful things He has done in your life. Soak in His love. Review the many ways you can spend time with God, enjoying His presence and your time with Him. Get alone with God right now and try the new way of showing joy in your relationship with him, the way you circled on Day 5. You'll find that praising your Lord and Savior, who loves you so much, provides greater enjoyment than eating food or giving in to a temptation!

> *Lord, I desire a relationship with You more than I desire anything else. Help me pursue You with the same energy I pursue other forms of joy. Amen.*

REFLECTION AND APPLICATION Day 7

> *Dear Lord, I am amazed that You, the Ruler of the universe, want a relationship with me! But I believe Your Word, which says that if I draw close to You, You will draw close to me. Teach me what is best for me. Amen.*

When you're reading and studying God's Word, talking to Him in prayer, listening to His response through the Holy Spirit, and putting His commands into practice in your daily life, you're having a spiritual relationship with God.

Consistency and frequency are key to a fulfilling spiritual life, and like any two-way relationship, you must contribute to keeping it alive and vibrant. Just as you don't feast one day and fast for weeks, living on the memory of your last delicious meal, you can't live on the memory of an occasional wonderful time with the Lord and expect to have a growing spiritual life.

Satan doesn't want you having a relationship with God, and he'll do everything in his power to thwart your spiritual growth. Oh, the excuses will seem real enough—but consider the source of the sudden headache the morning of Bible study group, that project deadline requiring you to work on Sunday, the fight with a child or spouse on the way to church, sleeping through the alarm after you had decided to get up early and have a quiet time with God.

You have to *make* time for God, or it isn't going to happen. Prayerfully put on the armor of God in the morning and cast off every arrow that Satan sends to thwart your best intentions of developing your spiritual relationship with God throughout the day.

A daily quiet time is a great start, but a meaningful relationship that truly brings joy requires ongoing two-way communication. Too often, our spiritual life is relegated to a few stolen moments, and we wonder why we're stumbling in our walk with the Lord. Two-way communication should take place throughout the day, especially when you're tempted in some way to make an unhealthy choice.

Ask for forgiveness and for God to show you ways to ensure that nothing gets in the way of your time with Him. Here's a suggestion to get you started. You have a daily food plan, so now construct a daily "enjoying God plan." In the following chart, indicate the time each day when you will meet with God, and predetermine what you will do. This might mean replacing things that you should remove or limit in you life anyway. Be creative, such as listening to Christian radio stations or CDs while walking or driving.

Time	Enjoying God's Plan						
	Sun.	Mon.	Tue.	Wed.	Thu.	Fri.	Sat.
Morning							
Noon							
Afternoon							
Evening							

It takes three weeks to break a habit and three weeks to start a new one, but you'll find spending time with the Lord is so enjoyable that you won't be counting!

Lord, thank You for Your patience with me. I praise You, Father, that You never give up on me. Thank You for returning to me. Amen.

Notes

1. Warren Wiersbe, quoted in Chris Tiegreen, *The One Year Walk with God Devotional* (Wheaton, IL: Tyndale House Publishers, 2004), October 25.
2. Charles Swindoll, quoted in Chris Tiegreen, *The One Year Walk with God Devotional* (Wheaton, IL: Tyndale House Publishers, 2004), October 28.
3. J. Edwin Orr, "Playing the Good News Off-Key," *Christianity Today* (January 1, 1982), pp. 24-25.

Group Prayer Requests

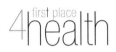

Today's Date: _____

Name	Request

Results

_____

_____

_____

_____

_____

_____

God's best for your circumstances

SCRIPTURE MEMORY VERSE
Give thanks in all circumstances, for this is God's will for you in Christ Jesus.
1 THESSALONIANS 5:18

Life consists of moments, occasions, incidents and circumstances—few of which we can control and all of which are the result of other people's right or wrong actions and choices (or our own). We try maintaining an environment of our choice, but the truth is that much of life happens around us, through us, for us—without so much as a nod in our direction, much less a handover of the control. Even so, we often fall into the "if only" or "when" trap, where we're sure that we would be happy and grateful *if only* our circumstances were different or that we will be happy and grateful *when* our circumstances are different. "If only" and "when" rationalizations cause many people to miss the joy of the present.

Use this opportunity to discard any "if only" and "when" myths that have a grip on you. Write them below in the left-hand column:

"If only" or "when"	What you could change / be satisfied with

Take a few minutes to think about the list you just made. Now, in the right-hand column, tell either what you could do to help bring about the change you would like to see or why you could be satisfied with the way things are.

When we give our life to Christ, we allow Him to take control over our life—all the moments, occasions, incidents and circumstances. We think, *Not my way Lord, but Your way. Even when I don't understand everything, I trust You.* The Christian life means dying to self and being reborn in Christ and His ways. The Christian walk is a long, ongoing process as we strive for maturity, and it may take a lifetime to truly let go and let God. But no matter where we are on our walk with God or what our circumstances, we should always remember to be thankful.

Day 1

GIVE GOD THE GLORY

Lord, I often forget You are in every circumstance of my life. Nothing eludes You. Whether I think things are going well or poorly, remind me to thank You for my many blessings and not just come to You with a list of problems and requests. You are a good and gracious God. All things come from You. Amen.

When a pastor gives a sermon on this week's memory verse, "Give thanks in all circumstances, for this is God's will for you in Christ Jesus," we expect to hear about giving thanks in the midst of a crisis or tragedy. Some thesauruses even offer the words "accident" and "incident" as synonyms for "circumstance." But unhappy times are just one aspect of the verse. We also are to give thanks in the good and ordinary times of life—promotions, successful careers, great family, financial stability, good health.

These comprise "all circumstances" as much as loss of work, unstable career, broken family, bankruptcy, failing health. Naomi and Ruth endured difficult circumstances, but God brought good out of their hard times and He received the glory (see Ruth 2:20; 4:14). In the table on the following page, list Naomi and Ruth's circumstances and find the corresponding purpose each had in fulfilling God's plan.

Naomi's and Ruth's circumstances		God's purpose and plan
1:3-5	Naomi's husband and sons die	Naomi returns to her home in Judah
1:14-16		
2:1-3		
2:5-7		
3:1-4		
3:12		
4:13		

When we're in trouble, we cry out to God and plead for help, but when He answers, do we stop and say, "thank You"? Instead, *we* may take the credit for our good fortune, or we may attribute it to luck. When we don't attribute our good circumstances to God, we become prideful. Read 2 Corinthians 12:7-10. What did Paul mean when he wrote that he had a "thorn in my flesh"?

_____

_____

_____

What was God's response to Paul's pleading to have the thorn removed (see verse 9)?

_____

_____

_____

How did Paul respond to his circumstance (see verses 9-10)?

_____

_____

_____

Our memory verse for this week, 1 Thessalonians 5:18, is actually a warning: God will humble us if we think too highly of ourselves. When we don't give God the glory and honor that is due to Him, we sin. That may sound shocking, but it's true. Read Psalm 10:4-6 and fill in the missing words:

In his _____ the _____ does not seek him; in all his thoughts there is no room for God. His ways are always prosperous; he is _____ and your laws are far from him; he sneers at all his enemies. He says to himself, "Nothing will shake me; I'll always be _____ and never have trouble."

According to Proverbs 16:18, what will happen if we become prideful?

_____

_____

_____

_____

_____

Turn to Psalm 25:9. What does God promise for those who humbly give God the glory for their successes and happiness:

He [God] _____ the humble in what is right and teaches them _____

_____.

Every believer is seeking to know the right thing to do and to learn our Lord's ways. The answer to our quest is straightforward: Humbly thank God for who He is and the things He has done and will do! He will guide us and teach us as we continue to seek Him.

Father, there isn't enough paper in the world to put in writing my many blessings. I promise to start my prayers with gratitude for who You are and for what You have done. Thank You for Your grace and for picking me up when I fall. Thank You! Thank You! Thank You! Amen.

WHY ME? Day 2

Lord, being Your follower isn't always easy, and there are times I don't understand why You let me endure hardships. But help me to lean on You and not on my own understanding (see Proverbs 3:5). Amen.

When the bottom is falling out of our world, our first thought isn't usually, Thank You, Lord, for this new crisis! Usually our first words are, "Help me!" Or like the psalmist we may ask, "Why, O Lord, do you stand far off? Why do you hide yourself in times of trouble?" (Psalm 10:1).

On occasion, we've all asked God, "Why me?" Briefly describe one or two "Why me?" times in your life.

_____

_____

_____

The apostle Paul, the author of today's memory verse, certainly encountered circumstances in which he could have easily asked, "Why me, Lord? I'm only trying to serve You and spread the gospel." No one would have faulted him, but he never complained—not even when he developed the thorn in his side or during any of the other difficult circumstances he faced. Read 2 Corinthians 11:23-31. What hardships did Paul incur in his ministry (see verses 23-29?

_____

_____

_____

Even with the long list you just made, what does Paul say he boasts about (see verse 30)?

_____

_____

Paul knew that God could have prevented all of his difficult circumstances, but instead of blaming God, how did he respond (see verse 31)?

_____

_____

_____

Paul wasn't praising God *for* all the hardships, but *in* the midst of those dreadful circumstances the gospel was spread, and for that he was grateful: "For this is God's will for you in Christ Jesus." Look up Philippians 4:11-13. How did Paul endure his circumstances?

_____

_____

_____

Have you ever said, "I couldn't have made it through without the Lord"? You were right: you couldn't. Neither could Paul or anyone else in the Bible who experienced incredibly hard times in the name of the Lord. Read Proverbs 3:5 and Psalm 42:5. Who do we lean on? According to David, even though in our humanness we may feel sad or frustrated, what keeps us going?

_____

_____

_____

Like Paul and David, we must still praise God in difficult circumstances and put our hope in Him, because hope is confident expectation that God is in control when we know that we aren't.

Lord, I rest in the hope that comes from knowing You will never leave me or forsake me. Even when I don't see the answer, You have everything under control and You want only what is best for me. Amen.

WHY NOT ME?

Lord, I know You are directing my life and You have a plan. Help me live according to Your eternal purpose. Amen.

Yesterday we talked about "Why me?" Today, we'll look at "Why not me?" This was Job's response to his wife when she asked why he still had his integrity after the terrible things that happened to him: "Shall we accept good from God, and not trouble?" (Job 2:10). Experiences in a believer's life aren't random: God is sovereign and He has a plan and a purpose for our every circumstance.

Read Jeremiah 29:1-14. The Israelites' refusal to follow God's plan and the hardening of their hearts toward Him resulted in their exile. What did God tell the people to do while they were in exile (see verses 4-9)?

_____

_____

_____

How long was their circumstance going to last (see verse 10)?

_____

_____

_____

What was God's plan for them (see verse 11):

_____

_____

_____

What condition did God put on fulfilling His plan and purpose for them (see verses 12-14)?

_____

_____

Now look up James 1:2-4. How would the Israelites' experience mature them? What was God trying to achieve in their lives?

_____

_____

_____

_____

Turn to Romans 5:1-5. God cares more about our character than our comfort, and He will leave us in a circumstance until we seek Him with *all* of our heart and are transformed into the person who can achieve His purpose for our life. Describe this process and the end result (see verses 3-5).

_____

_____

_____

During our refining time, God watches to see if we live a life that reflects the hope found in a relationship with Jesus Christ. What are some of the signs that we still have hope in the midst of a difficult time?

_____

_____

_____

That brings us to Romans 8:28-29. Paul states that "in all things," just as "in all circumstances," God works in the lives of believers. Even though His "good" may not feel good to us, what is God's ultimate goal for us?

_____

_____

_____

Jesus, help me to see Your face shining through the difficulties of my day.
Help me to change my character, and continue to refine me, so I can better
serve You. Help me live according to Your plan for my life. Amen.

SOMEBODY'S WATCHING

Jesus, I want my walk to match my talk, and I pray that my life will be a good witness to my belief in You. Amen.

Not every circumstance is for our own character-building experience. Often God wants to use us as a witness to show others how a Christian deals with life. Study each situation in the following Scriptures and indicate whether the main character(s) was a good or bad witness for God.

Scripture	Good or bad witness?
Gen. 12:10-20	
2 Sam. 11:1-5	
Dan. 6:3-5	
Jon. 1:1-17	
Acts 16:22-34	

Fortunately, the biblical characters with a bad witness also had times of being a good witness. It's comforting to know we don't have to be perfect, but we need to be aware that people could be turned away from God based on our behavior. How was Naomi a good witness to Ruth?

_____

_____

_____

Read in Mark 2:1-12, a familiar story of a seemingly impossible circumstance. What motivated the men who carried the paralytic (see verse 5)?

_____

_____

_____

The four men were probably focused on helping their paralyzed friend, but while they carried him down the street, took him up to the roof, dug a hole in the roof and lowered him down to Jesus, who witnessed their act of faith (see verses 6-7,12)?

_____

_____

_____

What was the response of others who witnessed the results of these men's faith (verses 7,12)?

_____

_____

_____

The four men didn't say to their friend, "There's a great healer down the street. Too bad He doesn't come to your house to heal you." And they didn't say, "We know of a great healer, but it wouldn't make any difference if He saw you because your situation is impossible." They had a faith that didn't back away, and God's work was accomplished, not only for the physical and spiritual healing of the paralytic, but also for the benefit of the observers. Describe a time when you helped someone in trouble. Did you worry about how much time your help would take?

_____

_____

_____

Think of three spiritually paralyzed co-workers, friends or family members who are likely to see you often enough that they would be able to observe how you respond to your circumstances. Write their names and make a commitment to God and yourself to be a witness who draws them closer to God.

1. _____

2. _____

3. _____

*Dear God, I want my life to be a witness for You. Please give me the words
I need to share with others that the source of my hope is You. Amen.*

HOW DO YOU SAY THANKS? Day 5

*Dear Lord, help me be a happy person with my perspective
on heaven and not on the worries of this world. Teach me to pray,
"Your will be done on earth as it is in heaven." Amen.*

You've seen them—the happy people who praise their Savior regardless
of the circumstances. How can these people find joy in the midst of pain
and loss, or smile when everyone else expects a frown? These people do
experience sadness, but they also understand that God's best for their life
is for them to give thanks in all earthly circumstances. When you know
that you will be spending eternity in paradise with Jesus Christ, you can
smile through your tears.

God wants us joyfully praising Him—with our whole heart, soul and
mind—regardless of the circumstances, because being "in Christ Jesus,"
we cherish, love and trust Him. Psalm 55:17 assures us that whenever
we cry out to God, "he hears [our] voice." God uses our distress to help
us grow. Because of that fact, some people look at distressful times as a
blessing, because those times cause a transformation in their spiritual
life or the lives of others who see how they react to the bad times.

Many of David's psalms were mournful cries to God for help, because
David knew that only God could turn his mourning into joyful danc-
ing again. Read Psalm 30:10-12. How does this passage encourage you to
apply our memory verse in your own difficult circumstances?

_____

_____

_____

David composed Psalm 34 while running from King Saul who was trying
to kill him. Instead of lamenting to God about how unfair and unjustified

his circumstances, David sang praises to God for saving his life. David focused on the blessing of *refuge,* instead of the emotion of *rancor:*

I will extol the Lord at _____ _____; his praise will _____ be on my lips (v. 1). Those who look to him are _____; Their faces are never covered with _____ (v. 5). _____ and see that the Lord is _____; _____ is the man [or woman] who takes refuge in him (v. 8).

Now turn to Psalm 69:1-5. Things weren't going well for David when he wrote this psalm either, but regardless of his dire circumstances, what does David still do (see verse 30)?

_____

_____

_____

_____

The Bible says to praise God "at *all* times"—when you feel like it and even when you don't. How can you do that? Read 1 Thessalonians 5:16-18. Paraphrase these verses in such a way that the three instructions in these verses lead one to the next.

_____

_____

_____

_____

Read Psalm 100, known as "A Psalm for Giving Thanks." How is Psalm 100:1 similar to 1 Thessalonians 5:16; and how is Psalm 100:4-5 similar to 1 Thessalonians 5:17-18?

_____

_____

_____

_____

God never moves, but we may distance ourselves from Him. Briefly describe a time you felt distant from God while being battered and discouraged by a circumstance. How could the prescription in Psalm 100 and 1 Thessalonians 5:16-18 have helped you enter into God's presence again?

_____

_____

_____

Thank You, Lord, for reminding me that my joy doesn't depend on my circumstances. Help me find my happiness in knowing You love me. Amen.

REFLECTION AND APPLICATION

Day
6

Lord, I often feel so small and insignificant and can't imagine that You could have a purpose for me. But because I believe Your Word, I will do great things for You when given the opportunity. Amen.

The story is told that many years ago, a large American shoe manufacturer sent two sales reps out to different parts of the Australian outback to see if they could drum up some business among the Aborigines. Some time later, the company received telegrams from both agents. The first one said, "No business here. Natives don't wear shoes." The second one said, "Great opportunity here—natives don't wear shoes."

In the Chinese language, the word for "crisis" is a combination of two characters—one meaning "danger" and the other, "opportunity." Many circumstances can actually be opportunities, depending on your perspective and whether you've developed an attitude of gratitude. Look back at this week's introduction, where you listed our "if onlys" and "whens." See if you can say, "Thank You, Lord, for this situation, just as it is. I will look at this situation as an opportunity to effect a change in my life. For each one that you can say that about, write, "Thank You, God," next to it.

Then, every morning, pray, "God, how can You use me today in the midst of my circumstances?" Write the word "Opportunity" on an index card and use it for a bookmark in this study as a reminder to apply what you're studying to enrich your life and the lives of others. Look for opportunities to be a light in a dark world, where many people are taking drastic measures to relieve their pain.

Lest you think only the great people of the Bible could truly thank God for everything that came into their life, read a praise report from a woman being treated for stage three ovarian cancer whose husband fell off a ladder and incurred a compression fracture of his T-11 vertebra, collarbone and rib: "We truly are praising God for the angels that were attending Jim even as he fell! And we're thanking God for all the medical staff, who cared for him once the fracture was discovered, on through the surgery, and into recovery!"

That quote is from a missionary couple, mature in their faith and grounded in the Word. When they were put under pressure, they displayed their faith. You don't have to be a missionary to possess that kind of faith; you just need to "give thanks in all circumstances, for this is God's will for you in Christ Jesus." God has a purpose in all your pain. He can use unhappy circumstances to mature you and can use your positive reactions to unhealthy circumstances to bring unbelievers close to Him. The test of your faith isn't in the good times but when the tough times come. Keep growing in your spiritual life—that is God's best for all life's circumstances.

Lord, I know it will be a challenge for me to praise You in all circumstances, but I do pray that thanksgiving exudes from me in difficult times. With Your strength, joyful praise will become my natural response in all circumstances.

Day 7

REFLECTION AND APPLICATION

Your love is so amazing, Father. I will be glad and rejoice in it, even when my circumstances are not as I desire. Help me to bloom where I'm planted. Amen.

Barbara Ann Kipher began keeping a list of her favorite things when she was a teenager. Soon the list became second nature and she found herself making additions to the list in *all* circumstances of her life: riding the bus, eating breakfast and even in the middle of the night. Twenty years and dozens of spiral notebooks later, her list was published as a book titled *14,000 Things to Be Happy About*.

You could also write a book in the form of a prayer and praise journal. Start by recording how God answers your question from yesterday—how He can use you in the midst of your circumstances—and record the results of your actions of faith. You will have a record of God at work in your life.

You also can journal your daily prayer requests and give thanks to God for how He answers. Often, it is easy to forget that we asked God for something. Our circumstances change or get better, and we give everyone the praise except the Lord. Keeping a prayer and praise journal will remind you to give thanks, and it will also be a legacy of God at work in your life.

Take a journal or, like Ann Kipher, a spiral notebook, and three quarters across on each page draw a vertical line to make a column. Head the first column "prayer requests" and the second column "praises." Journal your daily prayers, and at the end of each week, reread your requests and note in the praise column how God has answered it. Always put a "thank You" to God, regardless of whether it was the response you wanted. God answered in the way He knew was best for you, even if the answer happened to be "wait."

Close this week's study by writing a thank you card to God for a circumstance in your life that drew you closer to Jesus. Keep the card in your Bible so that when troubles come—and they will—you can read your card and feel the gates of His presence opening as you enter in worshipful praise.

Lord, the Bible is a record of Your legacy, and I want to have
a record of what You have done in my life. Help me remain
faithful to recognizing You in the midst of this crazy life, and let
me leave a legacy that displays You at work in my life. Amen.

Group Prayer Requests

4health first place

Today's Date: _____

Name	Request

Results

_____

_____

_____

_____

_____

_____

God's best for your waiting rooms

SCRIPTURE MEMORY VERSE

While we wait for the blessed hope—the glorious appearing of our great God and Savior, Jesus Christ, who gave himself for us to redeem us from all wickedness and to purify for himself a people that are his very own, eager to do what is good.

TITUS 2:13-14

We spend much of our life waiting—for the doctor to see us, for the movie to start, for the light to change—yet most people detest waiting. Our natural impatience with waiting intensifies proportionately with the technological advances in this electronic age.

We live in a microwave, instant messaging, instant pudding, instant replay, fast-food, drive-thru, email, texting, twittering, ATM era. We are a generation obsessed with speed, yet our mantra is, "I don't have enough time."

Still, there remains a great number of things on God's timetable that we can't speed up: the full development of a baby in a mother's womb; a seed sprouting, growing and flowering; the amount of exercise required to lose a pound; the rising and setting of the sun and moon; the days in a week; the hours in a day; and our "blessed hope" the day of Jesus Christ's return to earth.

It could be a long wait, or Jesus could return even before you finish doing today's study. What a sobering thought. Even more sobering, though, is that we wait as a redeemed people who represent the Lord Jesus Christ.

WAITING FOR THE DAY

*Lord, it's the unknown element of waiting that's so hard. I'm good at waiting,
and I waste time and energy worrying while I wait. Help me learn patience.*

Think back to yesterday and record every occasion when you waited for
something or someone. What did you wait for? (Include things like waiting for the alarm to go off, waiting for your food to heat up, waiting in
line at the store). How long did you wait? What did you do while waiting?

What you waited for	Time waited	Activity while waiting

Total up the number of minutes you waited, divide it by your waking
hours, and you'll have the percentage of your day spent waiting. How
could you make your waiting time more productive?

_____

_____

_____

Think of all the physical, mental, emotional and/or spiritual issues for
which you are waiting for a resolution. (Include things like waiting for
a big deal to close, waiting to lose five pounds, waiting to get pregnant—
you get the idea.) How are you handling the wait?

Life's waiting rooms	How I'm handling the wait

While waiting in our daily lives, we may lose sight of the most important wait of our life—Jesus' return! Read Luke 12:35-48 to learn what Jesus said about His coming back. How should we wait (see verses 35-38)?

_____

_____

_____

When will Jesus come (see verses 38-40)?

_____

_____

What should we do while we wait for Jesus' return (see verses 42-44)?

_____

_____

_____

What happens if we get impatient and lose hope (see verses 45-47)?

_____

_____

_____

Why is more expected of a believer than an unbeliever (see verse 48)?

_____

_____

_____

How does the reality that *today* could be *the day* change your perspective in regard to your current "waiting rooms"?

_____

_____

_____

_____

Dear Jesus, forgive me for worrying about the inconvenience of my daily waiting rooms instead of focusing on Your imminent return. Help me live each day in light of eternity. Amen.

MENTORING AND BEING A ROLE MODEL

Dear Father, there is so much information available in my world. How can I decipher the good from the bad—what is Your will and Your way and not just my will or the world's way? Teach me to be more discerning. Amen.

In light of eternity, our earthly life is a God-given moment of opportunity to make a difference in this world before being transported to our permanent heavenly home. While we wait, God prepares us for the work we are to do while we're here. But waiting is very difficult, and sometimes we get tired and discouraged. When we lose sight of what we're eagerly awaiting, the waiting can turn to drudgery, which soon turns to disappointment, which eventually spirals downward into defeat. That's why we need another believer to come alongside us and remind us of our redemption, saved for God's purpose "to do what is good."

The memory verse this week comes from a letter Paul sent to Titus, a young disciple with whom Paul had introduced Christianity to the city of Crete. Titus was to organize the converts and teach them how to set up a church (see Titus 1:5). What was Paul's warning to Titus (see Titus 1:10-16)?

_____

_____

_____

Since there were false teachers in town, new Christians needed to know the truth, so Paul outlined a mentoring plan. Read Titus 2:1-8. What were the spiritually older men and women to do with what Titus taught them?

_____

_____

_____

Spiritual mentoring involves a spiritually older believer coming alongside a spiritually younger believer and being a role model of the Christian life. How did Naomi mentor Ruth (see Ruth 3:1-4,16-18)?

_____

_____

_____

Our memory verse is part of a detailed description of what Christians should be taught. Read Titus 2:11-15. Who can receive God's grace and salvation (see verse 11)?

_____

_____

_____

What should mentors teach regarding how Christians live under God's grace (see verses 12,15)?

_____

_____

_____

Why is it possible for us to live pure lives (see verses 13-14)?

_____

_____

_____

If you're a new Christian, having a spiritually older mentor is essential. Perhaps someone in your First Place 4 Health group or in your church could mentor you. Remember that there are many false teachers ready to educate you in the world's ways (see Revelation 12:9), so don't be fooled!

Lord, teach me Your ways and bring a godly mentor into my life to be a role model of the Christian life for me. Once I've learned to live a balanced life pleasing to You, I'll look for opportunities to teach and mentor others. Amen.

Day 3 — EAGER TO DO GOOD

Jesus, I know good from bad and right from wrong, but sometimes I'm not as eager as I should be to do the right thing. Help me put worldly things aside and only do things that are right in Your sight. Amen.

There is a difference between knowing what is good and eagerly doing it. We know going to church is good, but do we go with eager anticipation or reluctant duty? We know that eating healthy food is good, but do we eagerly eat nutritious food? We know that exercise is good, but are we always eager to get the blood pumping?

Yesterday, we looked at Titus 1:10-16, where Paul warned Titus about false teachers claiming to know God but denying Him by their actions. According to verse 16, these false teachers:

> Claim to _____ _____, but by their _____ they deny him. They
> are _____, _____ and _____ for doing anything good.

Ouch! That's a harsh statement, but it's a wake-up call to all Christians. We've all heard the adage "Actions speak louder than words," but while we're in our waiting rooms, do our actions shout what we *say* we believe about God? If we turn to the world's disobedient ways, what does our behavior convey?

_____

_____

_____

_____

Christians are to follow Jesus' example of "doing good" (Acts 10:38). In Titus 2–3, Paul instructs us in several ways on how we can "do good" for others. In the chart of the following page, list what Paul instructs in each passage of Scripture.

Scripture	How we can "do good" for others
Titus 2:3	
Titus 2:7	
Titus 2:12-13	
Titus 3:1-2	
Titus 3:9	
Titus 3:14	

Jesus used many parables to impress His followers with the importance of doing good and to define the good He wanted them to do. Turn to Matthew 25:14-30 and read the parable of the talents. What good did the man want his servants doing with the talents He had given them (see verses 15-17,19-23)?

_____

_____

_____

_____

What was the consequence for the servant who was afraid to use his talent and buried it (see verses 26-29)?

_____

_____

_____

_____

Originally "talent" referred to a unit of weight and later to a coin, but today what does "talent" mean?

_____

_____

_____

_____

What are your God-given gifts and talents, and how *eagerly* are you using them for the Lord?

_____

_____

_____

Who sets the example for eagerly doing good, and who will empower you to go and do the same (Acts 10:38)?

_____

_____

_____

> *Lord, thank You for the gifts and talents You've given me. Open my eyes for opportunities to use them to do good for Your glory. Amen.*

Day 4

WISDOM WAITS

Dear God, too often I'm impatient and I think I know what to do, so I don't stop to receive wise counsel or wait on Your leading and direction. Teach me to be still and wait on You. Amen.

Chris Tiegreen states, "Wisdom is a right understanding of the world and our role in it. It knows who God is, it knows who we are, and it sees the relative importance of all things. It is a correct ordering of priorities, majoring on truth and character before superficial pleasers. It is the only way, in the long run, to be truly satisfied."[1] Read Proverbs 3:5-8 and Proverbs 4:6-8. What value does wisdom have?

_____

_____

_____

How can we seek God's wisdom (see Proverbs 4:1-5)?

_____

_____

_____

God's plan for us may involve waiting for a future resolution to a problem or our waiting as a test of our faith. Often we can't imagine why He would want us waiting at all, so we impulsively take action to achieve the most expedient, visible and least-painful solution to whatever problem we are facing. What does the Bible call us, and what can be the results, when we act on our own understanding or what seems like the logical and natural thing to do (see Proverbs 16:25; 18:2; 1 Corinthians 1:20-21)?

_____

_____

_____

King David wrote many mournful waiting psalms, and there were times when he didn't wait or listen to wise counsel—with dreadful results. Read 2 Samuel 24:2-17. What did David impulsively do, and what were the consequences (see verses 2-4,13-15)?

_____

_____

_____

God is never in a hurry. The Scriptures don't describe any time when He was indecisive, panicked, impulsive or searching for answers. God is sovereign over all things and is looking over our situation and into the future. This concept is so difficult for us to comprehend that the Bible repeatedly reinforces it. Read Psalm 27:14 and fill in the blanks:

_____ for the Lord; be strong and take heart and _____ for the Lord.

Do you ever find it hard to wait? Do you ever try to rush ahead of God? If so, why do you think that is the case?

_____

_____

_____

How can we hear God clearly (see Psalm 46:10)?

_____

_____

_____

The following acrostic is based on Psalm 13, written by King David who learned to wait for an answer from God, even when under siege; it might help you relax and wait on God's timing. Take one of your "waiting room" issues and apply this acrostic by writing what you will do in regard to your issue.

Watch God at work (see verse 3).
  I will _____
Ask God (see verses 1-2).
  I will _____
Invite God to join you (see verses 3-4).
  I will _____
Trust/Thank God (see verses 5-6).
  I will _____

Rest assured that you'll hear from God: "Whether you turn to the right or to the left, your ears will hear a voice behind you, saying, 'This is the way; walk in it'" (Isaiah 30:21).

Lord, If I trust and rest in Your Sovereignty, everything will turn out as You planned. Thank You, Father, for helping me to be wise in my waiting. Amen.

Day
5

GETTING READY

Jesus, I do savor the hope of Your return, and I want others to share my hope. Let me live ready to meet You at that hour when You take me home. Amen.

Are you ready for the glorious day when Jesus will return? Often we joke about the Rapture coming before we have to face major events, health problems or weight issues. But Jesus wants us in our best shape—emotionally, physically and spiritually—when He does return. His desire is to greet each of us with, "Well done, my good and faithful servant. You did the best you could with what I gave you. Good job!" Would you be ready to see Jesus face to face if He came back tonight? What, if any, changes would you want to make in your life, and what would you do to effect each change?

Changes to prepare for Jesus' return	What I will do to make that change

Sometimes we're fearful of Jesus' actual return. It's good to have a holy fear in anticipation, but letting go of this world will be a good thing, so we shouldn't be afraid. Read 1 John 2:15-17. What in this world might have an unhealthy hold on you?

_____

_____

_____

_____

Look up 1 Thessalonians 4:15-18. According to verse 18, what are we to do with this vital information?

_____

_____

_____

Read Hebrews 3:12-14. In what practical ways could you encourage your First Place 4 Health group, your friends and your family to live in ready anticipation of Christ's return?

_____

_____

_____

_____

Lord, I don't know what the day of Your return will be like, but I know that it will be magnificent. Help me make the changes that would honor You when we meet face to face on that glorious day. Amen.

Day 6 — REFLECTION AND APPLICATION

Dear Lord, during the times when I'm tempted to act impulsively and not wait for Your will to be done, please bring to my mind everything You have done for me. Teach me how to search for Your ways and Your will. Amen.

You might be enthusiastic about applying this week's lesson today, but as time passes and new trials, troubles and waiting rooms appear, you might find it easy to slip back into old patterns of taking matters into your own hands. Since the beginning of time, God's people have forgotten His faithfulness. During the time of the Old Testament, the Israelites repeatedly clung to God and followed His way only to eventually turn from Him, forget His promises and try to do things on their own.

When we do what *we* think is best without waiting for *God's* best, we operate under the limitations of our finite mind and resources. We often disparage the Israelites, but at times we are no different. We want to rush ahead of God and make things happen. God's response is worth the wait, but He can't come to those who won't wait.

Meditate today on Psalm 106—a recount of the rebellious, impatient Israelites, who repeatedly forgot that God *always* came through as their defender, deliverer, provider, protector and miracle worker, if only they would wait on His timing.

In Psalm 106:13, the psalmist says that the Israelites forgot God's counsel. Can you think of a time in your life when you didn't wait for the Lord's wise counsel? If so, describe the situation.

_____

_____

_____

_____

In verse 14, the psalmist says that the Israelites submitted to their cravings. How could submitting to your cravings be the result of not waiting on the Lord?

_____

_____

_____

_____

What has been the result of not following God's best in your "waiting rooms"?

_____

_____

_____

_____

How did God show His compassion to His people (see verses 44-46)? How has God shown His compassion for you?

_____

_____

_____

_____

Reflect on verses 14 and 47-48. When we forget how great our God is and the past rewards of waiting on Him, our discouragement and disappointment can result in surrendering to our cravings or addictions. Spend the rest of your time today praising your Lord and Savior and ask Him to remind you of everything He has ever done for you. As His blessings come to mind, write them down and post the list on your refrigerator.

> *Praise You, Lord. You never give up on me, even when it seems I've given up on You, Lord, You always wait for me. Forgive my impatience. I promise to slow down and look up. Amen.*

Day 7 — REFLECTION AND APPLICATION

Dear Jesus, You want the best for me, and that usually involves taking my focus off myself and focusing on serving You and others. I pray this concept will come more naturally to me than it does right now. Thank You for the reminder. Amen.

In the parable of the sheep and the goats in Matthew 25:31-46, Jesus made clear that the good we eagerly do here on earth is the same that we do for Him (see verse 40). In other words, when we show love to someone else, we are showing love to Jesus. Jesus spoke figuratively in His parable, of course, but what practical things could you do in the six areas that He listed?

Jesus' words	What I will do to make that change
"I was hungry and you gave me something to eat" (verse 35).	
"I was thirsty and you gave me something to drink" (verse 35).	
"I was a stranger and you invited me in" (verse 35).	
"I needed clothes and you clothed me" (verse 36).	

Jesus' words	What I will do to make that change
"I was sick and you looked after me" (verse 36).	
"I was in prison and you came to visit me" (verse 36).	

Now, pray over the list and determine the order you will do these good deeds—as if you were doing them for the Lord. As you serve and help others, notice how much better you feel about your own waiting rooms. What can you learn by serving others?

_____

_____

_____

_____

*Father, the first step in healing is helping, so the way to live
in my waiting rooms is to be a good witness to others through my actions
and my deeds. When others ask how I can remain so calm and patient, I'll
readily tell them that the source of my strength is You! Praise You, Lord,
for keeping me company in my waiting rooms. Amen.*

Note

1. Chris Tiegreen, *The One Year Walk with God Devotional* (Wheaton, IL: Tyndale House Publishers, 2004), February 26.

Group Prayer Requests

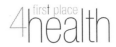

Today's Date: _____

Name	Request

Results

_____

_____

_____

_____

_____

_____

God's best for your appearance

SCRIPTURE MEMORY VERSE

The LORD does not look at the things man looks at. Man looks at the outward appearance, but the LORD looks at the heart.

1 SAMUEL 16:7

In an attempt to look and smell better, Americans spend more than 8 billion dollars a year on cosmetics and another 12 billion dollars on perfume or cologne. Not to mention what the dollar equivalent would be for all the time spent applying and removing cosmetics and time spent washing and styling hair! We've all contributed to the staggering dollar amounts, and there's nothing inherently wrong with wanting to improve or enhance our appearance or our scent. However, this week's memory verse is a startling reminder that we do this primping on our outer selves for us and others—loved ones and strangers alike—while God cares more about the condition of our inner appearance.

God's perfectly happy with us just the way He formed us: "fearfully and wonderfully" in our mother's womb (Psalm 139:14). What He's most concerned about is the time and effort we expend beautifying our inner soul, which outlives our earthly body. In the chart on the following page, list the beauty, skin care and hair products you regularly use and the approximate time involved in applying them daily. (If you're a man, think of colognes, shaving supplies and hair gel or hairspray). Total up the minutes or hours and compare that time with the total amount of time you spend with the Lord each day.

Cosmetic, skin care and hair products	Time spent applying	Time spent with the Lord

What did this exercise reveal to you?

_____

_____

_____

_____

Day 1

TRUE VALUES

Jesus, help me value what You value most. I'm always aware of how I look or how others are looking at me, but I want to concentrate on beautifying my inner self for an audience of One—You. Amen.

We've all seen elegantly dressed people greet each other with a pseudo kiss in the air, avoiding contact and not disturbing hair or makeup, while giving the once-over and gushing, "You look marvelous, darling!" The superficial gestures and insincere comments convey what each person is thinking: I'm really here to make an appearance, and I hope you aren't showing me up!

Our culture is exterior-oriented—physical appearance, homes, cars, schools, careers, income levels. Sadly, the same media sources influencing our culture also unveil the shallow, unfulfilling, empty and often tragic life of "the beautiful" people. Have you ever said, "She's so beautiful and thin, why would she engage in such damaging behavior?" Have you ever thought, *He has everything—why does he continue ruining his life with drugs, alcohol and sex?* The answer? Something vital is missing in their heart and soul that no amount of money, fame or beauty will satisfy. They're beautiful on the outside, but empty on the inside—rich, yet poor. There's a hole in their heart only Jesus can fill. You had that same hole before you gave your heart to Jesus and let Him fill it with the Holy Spirit.

Compare your life before and after accepting Jesus as your Savior. What were the major differences?

_____

_____

_____

_____

What are 10 things that the world values?

1. _____
2. _____
3. _____
4. _____
5. _____
6. _____
7. _____
8. _____
9. _____
10. _____

Read Luke 16:14-15. How does God feel about what the world values?

_____

_____

_____

_____

What the world considers important and valuable is the exact opposite of what God values. Let's look at things that are different on earth than in heaven. Read these verses from Matthew 5 and describe what the world values as opposed to what God values.

Verse(s)	What the world values	What God values
v. 3		
v. 5		
v. 6		
v. 10		
vv. 38-40		
v. 41		
v. 42		
vv. 43-44		

With which of these values do you struggle the most?

_____

_____

_____

Father, I have bought into the world's lies regarding what's valuable. My desire is to stay close to You and focus only on what's pleasing to You. Amen.

Day 2

HEART CHECK

I love You, Lord, with all my heart. Please help me have a godly countenance that reflects Jesus. Amen.

Many Scriptures, including this week's memory verse, talk about the heart. You know the heart is an organ in our physical body, and its health and condition is vital to sustaining human life; but did you know that the health and condition of your spiritual heart is essential to sustaining spiritual and physical life? Theologian Dallas Willard advises, "Put everything you have into the care of your heart, for it determines what your life amounts to."[1] You may find it difficult to know what's best for your life, but the Bible provides wise counsel for confidently knowing God's best.

Look up Psalm 119:9-12. To whose words should you pay close attention, and where should you keep those words?

How will keeping God's Word in your heart affect your body and life (see Proverbs 4:22-23)?

Christian discussions and the Bible frequently use the word "heart." In 1 Chronicles 28:9, King David explained the anatomy of a spiritual heart to his son Solomon:

> And you, my son Solomon, acknowledge the God of your father, and serve him with wholehearted devotion and with a willing mind, for the Lord searches every
> _____ and understands every _____ behind the
> _____. If you seek him, he will be found by you; but if you forsake him, he will reject you forever.

Complete the following sentence, filling in the blank with something you're trying to achieve for your appearance:

I have my <u>heart</u> set on _____.

According to 1 Chronicles 28:9, your heart is the axis of motives, which triggers thoughts and actions. In a dictionary or a thesaurus, find synonyms for "heart" and "motive" and write them below.

Synonyms for "heart"	Synonyms for "motive"

Now say aloud the sentence you completed above, replacing the word "heart" with the synonyms. What new insight into the significance of nurturing the spiritual condition of your heart have you found?

_____
_____
_____
_____

While the appearance of your face and body is visible to onlookers, who are the only two "in-lookers" who really know the appearance of your heart (see 1 Kings 8:38-39)?

_____
_____
_____
_____

According to the following Scriptures, how does God help you maintain a heart pleasing to Him?

1 Kings 8:58-62

_____

_____

_____

2 Chronicles 16:9

_____

_____

_____

Create in me a pure heart, O God, and renew a steadfast spirit within me (Psalm 51:10). Keep my motives honorable, my mind pure and my intentions honest. I'm committed to doing Your will in every area of my life. Amen.

UNIQUE YOU

Day
3

Lord, I'm not always happy with the way You made me, because I still sometimes judge myself by the world's standards. Help me understand Your plan and purpose for unique me. Amen.

God created each of us unique as a snowflake—no two are the same— but sometimes our goal is to look like an imaginary princess or prince. Often we're not happy or satisfied with the way God made us, but as we read in Psalm 139:13-16 (see Week One), God created every part of us according to His plan, and each of us is beautiful to Him. Yet you still may wish He had made you with straight or curly hair—smaller or larger feet—shorter or taller.

Some people put pictures of models or body builders on their re- frigerator with aspirations of looking like these professionals. Some have even resorted to extreme measures like plastic surgery to fulfill their hope for a perfect outward appearance. Most people understand with their mind that they are unique, but they protest their uniqueness in their heart. Maybe that's why David closed Psalm 139 with verses 23-24:

Search me, O God, and know my _____; test me and know my anxious
_____. See if there is any _____ way in me, and lead me in
the way _____.

Start today by doing what the above verses suggest: Ask God to search your heart—the keeper of motives and thoughts. Then write what the Holy Spirit reveals to you.

What about my appearance makes me anxious?

_____

_____

_____

How might my ways of dealing with this anxiousness be offensive to God?

_____

_____

_____

When I reach my weight goal, will I still wish I could change something else about my appearance? If so, why would this be the case?

_____

_____

_____

In what ways have you tried to change your appearance? What was the result of each attempt?

Ways I've tried to change my appearance	Results

What does Ecclesiastes 8:1 say will enhance your appearance?

_____

_____

_____

Who is your source of wisdom, and where does wisdom reside (see 1 Kings 10:24)?

_____

_____

_____

_____

With God's wisdom in your heart, you'll have the right motives and thoughts regarding every aspect of life. You joined your First Place 4 Health group to learn how to enhance your physical appearance (and every other area of your life) in a healthy and wise way. When you reach your ideal weight, be cautious not to sabotage your great accomplishment by focusing on another "imperfect" area of your appearance.

In closing today, read how Solomon described his beloved in Song of Songs 4:1-7. Beauty really is in the eyes of the beholder, and Jesus Christ is your beholder.

> _You are my beholder, Lord. I know in my head that I am attractive to You._
> _Help me know in my heart that is true. Let me bask in Your adoring love._

INNER BEAUTY Day 4

Abba, Father, You see me as gloriously and wonderfully made, but when I look in the mirror, I only see flaws. Help me see myself as You see me. Amen.

God has a standard of beauty that differs greatly from the world's perspective. Read the Scriptures below and list the characteristics that God truly values and deems beautiful.

Scripture	Characteristic that God values
Prov. 31:30	
Luke 18:14	
1 Pet. 3:3-4	

God values character and faith rather than physical appearance. It is this difference that is the context of this week's memory verse. God assigned the prophet Samuel to anoint a new king, because the reigning king, Saul, had disobeyed Him. God sent Samuel to Jesse's house with the instruction that God was going to choose one of Jesse's sons as the next king. Samuel was sure God would pick Jesse's oldest son, Eliab, who was tall and handsome like King Saul (see 1 Samuel 9:2; 10:23-24). Read 1 Samuel 16:7. What was God's explanation for not choosing Eliab?

Jesse paraded more sons in front of Samuel, but God rejected them all until Jesse brought in from tending sheep his youngest son, David. In 1 Samuel 16:12-13, how did the Lord respond when David appeared?

While David was handsome like his brothers, what factor caused God to decide David would be the one to replace Saul (see 1 Samuel 13:13-15)?

Nowhere in the Bible is Jesus' physical appearance recorded. We can only assume that His appearance was not remarkable or extraordinary, because none of the gospel writers noted anything special about His looks. Read Isaiah 55:8-9. Why do you think God picked a Messiah who didn't physically stand out from the crowd?

What did Ruth see in Boaz's character that overshadowed his outer appearance (see Ruth 2:13-23; 3:10,15-17)?

Describe a time when you erroneously judged someone by his or her appearance, and explain how memorizing 1 Samuel 16:7 will help prevent this from happening in the future.

Accepting that each of us is unique and that God focuses on our individual inner beauty doesn't mean that physical appearance is irrelevant. Why do you still need to care for your body with proper hygiene and appropriate dress, regardless of where you are in the weight-loss process?

You aren't trying to win anyone's favor by appearing beautiful, but you are trying to win everyone's heart for Christ by your character.

Lord, I confess I often look first at outward appearance and then make a judgment about a person before getting to know the person. Help me see each person's inner beauty as You do, and remove my critical spirit. Amen.

Day 5

WHAT'S TRULY IMPORTANT

Lord, I don't always consult You first when evaluating my appearance. I'm usually more concerned about the opinion of others. Help me remember my confidence comes from You alone. Amen.

In Matthew 6:25-33, Jesus challenges us not to focus on the material things of this world or be too overly concerned about the things of this life. What types of things does Jesus tell us not to worry about in verses 25-26?

_____

_____

_____

What analogies does Jesus use in this passage to describe how God provides for our needs?

_____

_____

_____

Why does Jesus say that we do not need to be concerned about material things (see verses 26-27)?

_____

_____

_____

What are we to seek instead? What will be the result when we stop pursuing these things and give control of our lives over to God?

_____

_____

_____

In Week Two, you learned that you were created by God and in God's image. Look up Deuteronomy 32:4 and Matthew 5:48. How are God and His works described?

_____

_____

_____

Since what the Bible says is true, what does this tell you about how you should be describing yourself?

_____

_____

_____

_____

Read 1 Thessalonians 5:10-11. What are some ways that your First Place 4 Health group members could help each other to focus on what is truly important in this life?

_____

_____

_____

Dear Lord, thank You for caring about me and providing all I need. Help me to always give my concerns to You. Thank You for making me in Your image. Help me to be worthy of such a privilege. Amen.

REFLECTION AND APPLICATION

Day 6

Father, I often look at the person before I look into the person. Because I do this, I think others do the same with me. Help me love others as You do, regardless of how they look on the outside. Amen.

In her book *Henry Martyn: Confessor of the Faith*, Constance Padwick offers the following description of missionary Henry Martyn:

His features were not regular, but the expression was so luminous, so intellectual, so affectionate, so beaming with divine charity, that no one could have looked at his features and thought of their shape or form—the outbeaming of his soul would absorb the attention of every observer.[2]

Here is an instance of a person's heart showing in his outward appearance and overshadowing the physical characteristics by which we usually judge others. Unfortunately, when we first meet a person, we tend to make a snap judgment about that person based on his or her physical appearance. Try the following experiment this week: When you meet someone new, see if you first (1) judge the person's character by his or her physical appearance, or (2) get to know the person's character before noticing their appearance. If you consistently judge by appearance first, try silently praying 1 Samuel 16:7 when meeting a new person. Ask God to give you eyes to see beyond physical appearance and into his or her heart. Record the results of your experiment in your journal, and continue the experiment, until the result is a change in how you look at and judge others.

God, it's going to take practice for me to avoid sizing up someone or making a critical assessment based on superficial elements of appearance. Help me not only to give grace to others but also grace to myself. Amen.

Day 7

REFLECTION AND APPLICATION

Precious Jesus, I want to look at people as you do, and I want people to see that I am following Your way. Help me not to concern myself with this world and its values, but to seek Your wisdom and rewards. Amen.

Think of our hearts as a tablet that's been written on during our lifetime. It is a journal of all the information we've ever received—past relationships, media news, forms of entertainment, everyday experiences, comments others made about us, comments we've made, what we've read in the Bible—everything.

Satan tries to write unlovely things on our heart tablet—and some-times we hand him the pen. Sometimes we accept the media's and society's expectations and values, forgetting what God values. Perhaps some of us have tried to create a heart dictionary of the world's definitions of beauty, glamour, success and happiness. In fact, if we could remove our spiritual heart and examine it, some of what's written there might appall us! Yet we have reason to rejoice, because everything written on your heart is in washable ink. The blood of Jesus Christ was shed so that our tablet could be wiped clean and the world's writings could be replaced with the writings of our Lord and Savior.

Take a few moments to review Luke 16:14-15 from Day One. Ask God to reveal the unhealthy and "detestable" things written on your heart and list them on the following scroll in pencil. Then pray over the list, and as God brings to mind a healthy replacement, erase the unhealthy notation and write the replacement in permanent red ink to remind you of the blood Jesus shed to allow this change.

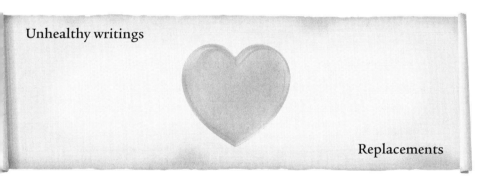

Unhealthy writings

Replacements

Dear Lord, this week has been revealing. Thank You for opening my eyes to what's really important. I pray I'll view others and myself as You do and not as the world does. I want to have Your Word in and on my heart. Amen.

Notes
1. Dallas Willard, quoted in Chris Tiegreen, *The One Year Walk with God Devotional* (Wheaton, IL: Tyndale House Publishers, 2004), March 11.
2. Constance E. Padwick, Henry Martyn: Confessor of the Faith (Chicago: Moody Press, 1980), p. 162.

Group Prayer Requests

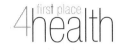

Today's Date: _____

Name	Request

Results

_____
_____
_____
_____
_____
_____

God's best for your attitude

SCRIPTURE MEMORY VERSE
Submit yourselves, then, to God. Resist the devil, and he will flee from you.
JAMES 4:7

Last week, we talked about the importance of determining the condition of our heart. What we find embedded there will manifest in either a good or bad attitude. Christian comedian Patsy Clairmont coined the phrase "sportin' a 'tude" to indicate a prideful, arrogant heart. This is the opposite of what the apostle Paul counseled Christians to reflect: the attitude of Christ and a humble heart (see Philippians 2:5,8).

If Jesus and His Word are the only residents in your heart, a bad attitude can't live there too. So, when you have a bad attitude, who has weaseled his way into your heart? You guessed it—Satan! Everytime you're sportin' a 'tude, Satan has moved in; and if you feel guilty for your 'tude, Satan unpacks his bags to stay. Now, don't start sportin' a 'tude that you'd never let Satan into your heart: pride hands him the key. This week we'll study how to resist the devil's attempts to invade your heart, so he'll flee before he even gets a chance to weasel his way in.

Dog lovers claim that you can tell a dog's attitude by its tail. If the dog's tail is wagging, he or she is in a playful, friendly mood. But if the dog's tail is standing straight up, beware. As we prepare to look at God's best for your attitude, take a moment and think about how people determine your attitude. How do you communicate "beware"? How do people know that everything is going great and you're happy?

To quote an old show tune, "You've gotta accentuate the positive [and] eliminate the negative."

LORD OF ALL

Dear God, You're Lord over everything. Why do I have trouble letting You be Lord over my life? I'm sorry for the times the devil shows through my attitude more than You do. Help me surrender all to You, Lord. Amen.

Our heart is the source of motivations, thoughts, emotions, intentions and beliefs—all of which influence our actions and attitudes. Whoever has a grip on our heart—the Lord or the devil—controls our attitude. What was Ruth's attitude in each of the following verses after her submission to God as her Lord?

Scripture	Ruth's attitude
Ruth 2:10-12	
Ruth 2:17-18	
Ruth 3:5	
Ruth 3:10-11	

If you've given your heart to Christ and made Him Lord of your life, how is it that you're occasionally sportin' a 'tude? That's what Paul asked the Colossians: "Since you died with Christ to the basic principles of this world, why, as though you still belonged to it, do you submit to its rules?" (Colossians 2:20). How would you answer Paul's question?

_____

_____

_____

Hudson Taylor wisely warned, "Christ is either Lord of all or He is not Lord at all."[1] Take a moment and prayerfully search your heart before answering this question: Have you submitted 100 percent of your heart to Jesus' lordship? If not, what part are you holding back, and why aren't you letting it go?

How could what you're hanging onto affect your attitude toward food, exercise and relationships?

Our memory verse this week cautions, "Submit yourselves, then, to God." Another word for "submit" is "surrender." Why do we naturally resist surrendering?

Read Romans 5-8. What happens to our relationship with God when we surrender, or submit, even partially to Satan?

Submission is not the same as obedience. We can *dutifully* but not *willfully*, obey. How does willingly offering yourself completely to God lead to *willful* obedience (see Romans 6:16)?

What do we gain from surrendering control of our lives to God?

Come to the_____ (2 Chronicles 30:8).

Submit to God and be at _____with him; in this way
_____ will come to you (Job 22:21).

How much more should we submit to the Father of our spirits and
_____! (Hebrews 12:9).

The rewards we gain from submitting ourselves to God are great, but the struggle against Satan is not an easy one. Charles Finney describes the struggle this way: "If you don't believe in the devil's existence, just try resisting him for a while."[2] This isn't an easy battle to win on your own, but you have the benefit of being in a group of like-minded people who will support each other in the battle. The rewards are so worth the fight!

Abba, there are times when my bad attitude is a reflection of the battle going on in my heart. I want to surrender 100 percent to Your lordship in my life, but it's hard for me to give up all control. Help me trust and obey. Amen.

Day 2 — WHAT'S IN AN ATTITUDE?

Lord, I often act like my attitude is my own business, but in my heart I know that isn't true. Please help me have an attitude that draws people to me. By having a good attitude, I'll also be drawing people to You. Amen.

A person's attitude doesn't go unnoticed, because it affects everyone around that person. Look up the word "attitude" in the dictionary. In what ways can a person display his or her attitude?

_____
_____
_____

A person's attitude usually either endears people or alienates them. What do the following Scriptures advise regarding God's best for your attitude?

Scripture	God's best for my attitude
Num. 12:3	
2 Sam. 9:6-7	
2 Chron. 30:22	
Prov. 25:15	
Matt. 19:19	
Heb. 13:1	

What is Satan's best for your attitude?

Scripture	Satan's best for my attitude
Ps. 94:3-5	
Prov. 16:18	
Prov. 25:14	
Prov. 29:22	
Isa. 46:12	
1 Cor. 4:18-19	

Read Proverbs 3:34. What is at the heart of negative attitudes? Positive attitudes?

_____

_____

_____

_____

Read Philippians 2:5-8. Whose attitude should we match, and what attributes of His attitude are we to emulate?

How would focusing on the interests of others and acquiring the humility of Christ Jesus change your attitude?

Jesus, You were perfect in every way when You humbled Yourself to come down to earth as a man. Lord, mold me and make me more like You. Amen.

Day 3

THERE'S GOING TO BE A TEST

Lord, You don't tempt me, but You do test my faith, and sometimes I don't pass the test. Help me maintain a faithful attitude that pleases You. Amen.

You're probably familiar with the SAT—Scholastic Aptitude Test—that measures students' knowledge before entering college. James, the author of this week's memory verse, has a SAT for believers—Spiritual Attitude Test—that measures the authenticity of faith and whether our behavior matches what we say we believe. Read Lamentations 3:40 and 2 Corinthians 13:5. What do these verses instruct us to do?

According to Hebrews 4:12, what should we use as the answer book to grade our SAT?

Take the following biblical SAT based on the book of James. What is your *usual* response when confronted by the following situations?

1. Face trials of many kinds: _____
2. Don't hear from God right away: _____
3. Lose at something: _____
4. Achieve success: _____
5. Are tempted: _____
6. Become angry: _____
7. Encounter people different from myself: _____
8. Hear of others in need: _____
9. Want what others have: _____
10. Experience suffering: _____

Next, for each question, look up the verse in James and write down the correct biblical response. Grade yourself using a scale of 1 (low—not even close) to 10 (high—just what the Bible says).

Scripture	God's best for my attitude
Jas. 1:2-4,12	
Jas. 1:5-7	
Jas. 1:9	
Jas. 1:10-11	
Jas. 1:13-18	
Jas. 1:19-21; 5:12	
Jas. 2:1-13	
Jas. 2:14-19	
Jas. 3:14-18; 4:1-6	
Jas. 5:7-11	

For each SAT question on which you scored low, commend yourself for being truthful! Then circle the correct responses for any situation in which you scored poorly. You might want to also consider listing these in your journal as a further reminder of where you need to improve. Of course, consistency in *inner* thoughts and *outer* actions equals integrity. When a person's mouth says one thing but his or her heart reflects something different, what did Jesus say that person should be called (see Matthew 23:28; Mark 7:6-7)?

_____

_____

_____

How did James describe people whose words don't match their actions (see James 1:22-25)?

_____

_____

_____

_____

As you take part in the First Place 4 Health program, test yourself often by questioning your attitude and your actions. Always make sure that your responses are biblical and healthy.

> *Father, I do believe in my heart that I can change offensive attitudes. Help me change my ways, Lord. Test me so I can come forth as pure as gold. Amen.*

Day 4 — ATTITUDE IS A CHOICE

Lord, I don't always take responsibility for how I act. Help me take ownership and responsibility for my actions. I want my behavior to please You. Amen.

Nothing can *make us* mad, *put us* in a bad mood or drive us crazy, but we love to fool ourselves and blame others or circumstances for our 'tude. This deception makes us feel that indulging in that extra scoop of ice cream, digging into a giant-sized candy bar, eating a whole pizza, going on a shopping spree or yelling at our kids or spouse is justified.

Viktor E. Frankl, a Nazi death camp survivor, recalled of his imprisonment: "Everything can be taken away from a man but one thing: the last of the human freedoms—to *choose* one's attitude in any given set of circumstances."[3] Although we can't control our circumstances, we can control our actions and reactions. We're in charge of our attitudes, and we make moment-by-moment choices.

Turn to Romans 7:15-24. What struggle did Paul have with his choices?

_____

_____

_____

Even when we *say* we don't want to do something, we, like the apostle Paul, often *choose* to keep on doing it anyway. In what areas are you experiencing the same struggle as Paul?

_____

_____

_____

A negative or discouraged attitude might result from unhealthy patterns developed over the years. Turn to Ephesians 4:22-24 to see what the Bible says about dealing with our past. What are we supposed to do about our old way of life—our old self (see verse 22)?

_____

_____

_____

How will this action affect our attitude (see verse 23)?

_____

_____

_____

What will our new self look like (see verse 24)?

_____

_____

_____

Being a Christian doesn't mean you won't be angry, sad, disappointed, frustrated. The choice you have, though, is whether you let these emotions fester and turn into actions that harm others or yourself. Read Romans 12:17-21. What problems can you *choose* to give to God right now?

_____

_____

_____

Choosing to have a good relationship with God means choosing to have a good attitude. If you're still struggling with your attitude, consider the fact that the problem may stem from not trusting in God's faithfulness. Personalize the following passage in Deuteronomy 31:8 by adding your name:

I know that the Lord Himself goes before _____ and will always be with _____; he will never leave _____ nor forsake _____.
I do not need to be afraid, and I do not need to feel discouraged.

Trusting in God's best for your life will change your attitudes and appetites.

Gracious God, help me find my identity in You and not in the world. I want to measure my worth solely by Your Word and live as Your righteous child.

Day
5

THE DEVIL HAS A 'TUDE

Oh, Lord, I haven't always resisted the devil like I should. Help me learn how to send Satan fleeing when his ugly presence interrupts my life. Amen.

This week's memory verse, James 4:7, promises us that if we resist the devil he will flee from us, but resisting isn't always easy. Or is it? Theologian, Jonathan Edwards summarized the Bible's answer to sending the devil on his way: "Nothing sets a person so much out of the devil's reach as humility."[4] Earlier this week, we established that pride is at the heart of many of our bad attitudes and that humility is its antidote. The disciple Peter concurred with James on how the devil uses our ego and pride to our own destruction. Both authors agreed that maintaining a humble, godly spirit and not submitting to the devil's cunning ways will send Satan packing. But he'll be back, and his favorite target is our "self."

Read 1 Peter 5:5-9. How will God help you maintain a humble attitude?

Where should you put concerns that negatively affect your attitude?

What is the only sure way to "resist the devil" (see 1 Peter 5:9)?

Read 1 Peter 3:10-12. Peter emphasizes the gravity of our role in making choices between good or evil by paraphrasing Psalm 34:12-16. What must people who "love life" do to "see good days"?

Daily we align ourselves with God or Satan. Allegiance to God must be a conscious choice. Use the following words to complete the formulas on the next page: allegiance, gratitude, action, praise.[5]

p _____ = an attitude of g _____

a _____ + alignment = attitude and a _____

Change doesn't happen on its own. How has participating in your First Place 4 Health group helped change your attitude in specific areas?

_____

_____

_____

As we close this week's lesson, read the prayer Paul sent to the church in Ephesians 3:17-20. Let it restore your resolve to stand firm in your allegiance to, and alignment with, Jesus Christ, who loves you too much to leave you the way you are.

Dear Jesus, I love You and I want Your best for me. Alert me to the devil's invasion of my attitude. I humbly ask forgiveness for the times I've let him influence me in the past and I ask for a renewed faith to resist him. Amen.

Day 6 — REFLECTION AND APPLICATION

Abba, Father, I admit that when I'm unhappy with myself, I'm not happy with anyone. Forgive me for the times my attitude has hurt someone, including myself. Help me love myself and others the way You do. Amen.

This week's emphasis was on attitude as a choice—*your* choice. The choice you make—and the attitude you have—is crucial to the success you have on earth and your relationship with God. Pastor Charles Swindoll recognized the significance of a person's attitude:

The longer I live, the more I realize the impact of attitude on life. Attitude, to me, is more important than facts. It is more important than the past, than education, than money, than circumstances, than failures, than successes, than what other people think or say or do. It is more important than appearance, giftedness or skill. It will make or break a company . . . a church . . . a home. The remarkable thing is we have a choice every day regarding the attitude we will embrace for that day. We cannot change our past. . . . We cannot change the fact that people will act in a certain way. We cannot change the inevitable. The only thing we can do is play on the one string we have, and that is our attitude. . . . I am convinced that life is 10% what happens to me and 90% how I react to it.[6]

The attitude we choose to display is a reflection of how we feel about ourselves. Eric Hoofer stated it beautifully when he said, "The remarkable thing is that we really love our neighbor as ourselves: we do unto others as we do unto ourselves. We hate others when we hate ourselves. We are tolerant toward others when we tolerate ourselves. We forgive others when we forgive ourselves. We are prone to sacrifice others when we are ready to sacrifice ourselves."

Last week you did a heart check. As you close this week, ask God to help you perform an attitude check. Think about how you perceive yourself, and then draw a line under those words that describe yourself.

Sassy	Polite
Critical	Forgiving
Bossy	Compassionate
Curt	Friendly
Aloof	Warm
Closed	Open
Negative	Positive

Now circle the words that describe how you think other people perceive you. Do your lines and circles always match up? Would Jesus be endeared or alienated by your attitude? Why?

_____

_____

_____

Pick a specific attitude you would like to change. Ask trustworthy friends, family members or First Place members to let you know when you're sportin' this 'tude. Then select a code word such as "ouch!" to use as a signal that your attitude needs improving. When you hear "ouch," immediately choose to change your attitude. Plan to make this attitude change permanent, and you'll eventually stop hearing "ouch!" Also notice whether people treat you differently when you practice a biblical attitude. Once you've mastered this attitude adjustment, move on to another attitude you would like to change. One day you'll wake up and, like Chuck Swindoll suggests, expertly play your "one string."

Dear Lord, if I publicly profess myself a Christian, I want to be the real deal. Please remind me when my attitude doesn't do You justice. Amen.

Day 7 REFLECTION AND APPLICATION

Dear Father, my bad attitude is my choice. Help me look at the brighter side of situations, by looking for Your purpose and plan. Help me turn lemons into lemonade, instead of displaying a sour attitude. Amen.

Much of our attitude is influenced by perspective: how we choose to look at someone or an event. In his book *Your Attitude: Key to Success*, John Maxwell shares the story of "Two Buckets": "There has never been a life as disappointing as mine," said the empty bucket as it approached the well. "I never come away from the well full, but what I return empty again." "There has never been such a happy life as mine," said the full bucket as it left the well. "I never come to the well empty, but what I go away again full."[7]

Think of a difficult situation with which you are currently dealing in your life. If you have a pessimistic bucket attitude, how would you approach the situation?

_____

_____

_____

If you have an optimistic bucket attitude, how would you approach the situation?

_____

_____

_____

_____

_____

Which approach was easier for you to describe? Which attitude has been your response up until now? If it was the negative, pessimistic attitude, ask God to change your 'tude. If you found it easier to write the optimistic approach, see if you can actually apply it to the problem you described.

Dear Jesus, You turn every opposition into an opportunity to further Your Kingdom here on earth. Help me learn to do the same. Today, I ask that You make me into a vessel that You can use for Your glory. Amen.

Notes

1. Hudson Taylor, quoted in Chris Tiegreen, *The One Year Walk with God Devotional* (Wheaton, IL: Tyndale House Publishers, 2004), February 28.
2. Charles Finney, quoted in Chris Tiegreen, *The One Year Walk with God Devotional* (Wheaton, IL: Tyndale House Publishers, 2004), October 18.
3. Viktor E. Frankl, *Man's Search for Meaning* (New York: Washington Square Press, 1984), p. 86.
4. Jonathan Edwards, quoted in Chris Tiegreen, *The One Year Walk with God Devotional* (Wheaton, IL: Tyndale House Publishers, 2004), October 18.
5. If you get stuck, the formula is "praise = an attitude of gratitude; action + alignment = attitude and allegiance."
6. Charles Swindoll, "Attitude," BigEye.com. http://www.bigeye.com/attitude.htm.
7. John C. Maxwell, *Your Attitude: Key to Success* (San Bernardino, CA: Here's Life Publishers, 1984), p. 22.

Group Prayer Requests

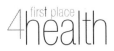

Today's Date: _____

Name	Request

Results

_____

_____

_____

_____

_____

God's best for your finances

SCRIPTURE MEMORY VERSE

My God will meet all your needs according to his glorious riches in Christ Jesus.
PHILIPPIANS 4:19

Our memory verse this week says that God will meet *all* our needs, and when we hear that promise, it's not surprising that we usually think of worldly material needs—the things that money can buy. But there's a qualifying second half to this verse we also must explore. God's best for your finances isn't only about money and what it can do for *you;* it's about all of your resources and how they can be used to further His kingdom.

Some people don't consider money an appropriate topic of conversation among Christians, unless the subject is tithing, financial counseling or the root of all evil. But money is the universal tool used worldwide to obtain goods and support and define lifestyles and cultures. Maybe we would tithe more, stay out of debt, and avoid wrongful uses of money if we had more teaching and training on God's best for our finances.

God talked about money, and there are more than 2,300 references to money and possessions in the Bible.[1] Out of the 38 parables Jesus told, 16 discuss how to handle money, and 1 out of every 10 verses in the Gospels refers to money or possessions. In fact, some scholars say that one-fifth of all Jesus said involved money.

Because a study of God's best for your life wouldn't be complete without a discussion of how money fits into your life, as a prelude to this week's study, briefly describe your financial situation.

_____

_____

_____

_____

NEED OR WANT?

Lord, as my Great Provider, You are aware of my every need, but I'm not always satisfied with Your provision. Help me learn to live within my means and be content with what You so generously give to me. Amen.

We start each morning "needy." We have routine needs (I need to get up), We have "should needs" (I need to lose weight), and we have "long for/crave/want needs" (I need a new car). Like a good parent providing for his children, our heavenly Father promises to supply all our *needs*—but not all our *wants*. Mankind has been in a tug-of-war with the Lord over needs versus wants since God created humans. In Week One, we learned how God provided all the survival needs of the first couple, Adam and Eve, who succumbed to the devil's sly introduction of a "long for" need, which became deadly. We scoff at Adam and Eve's foolish ungratefulness, but their story repeats itself throughout history. Do our houses, garages and storage units overflow with *needs* or *wants*?

Read Numbers 11:4-34. Take note of how the Israelites, God's precious people whom He loved, responded to God's provision for their survival. Then read the psalmist's interpretation of the Israelites' saga in Psalm 78:17-33. How did the Israelites sin against God, and what was God's response to their behavior (see Psalm 78:17-22)?

_____

_____

_____

How is manna described in Psalm 78:24-25 and in Psalm 105:40?

_____

_____

_____

How much manna were the Israelites to gather and what happened when they began hoarding it (see Exodus 16:4-5,16-20)?

_____

_____

_____

According to Psalm 78:25, God sent the Israelites "all the food they could eat," so why weren't they satisfied (see Numbers 11:4-6; Psalm 106:14)?

_____

_____

_____

What were the consequences of the Israelites testing God with their longings, cravings and wants, even though He provided for their daily needs (see Numbers 11:33; Psalm 106:15)?

_____

_____

_____

While providing for their current needs in the desert, God promised the Israelites "a land flowing with milk and honey" (Exodus 3:8). But because of their impatient wants and lack of trust in God's plan and provision, the Israelites wandered in the desert, eating manna for 40 years, and most missed receiving God's blessing—the Promised Land.

Naomi and Elimelech lived in the Promised Land, but fearing God wouldn't provide during the famine, they sought a better life in a pagan land and lost everything (see Ruth 1:21). When Naomi and Ruth returned to Judah 10 years later, who greeted Naomi, and what does that indicate about God's provision for the people who remained in Bethlehem (see Ruth 1:19)?

_____

_____

_____

Think about your own necessities for survival. How could you fulfill each category listed in the chart below? Indicate the fulfillment as a *need* and as a *want*. Follow the examples given.

Category	Need	Want
Food	*Healthy portions*	*Junk food*
Car	*Family or economy*	*Sports car*
Drink		
Income		
Clothes		
Entertainment		
Vacation		

My Father, You know what I need before I ask. Help me to discern the difference between a want and a need. Amen.

Day 2

WISDOM OR WEALTH?

Dear God, I want to be wise with all You've given me, and I want to trust that You always will provide whatever I need. Amen.

Advertising and marketing ploys designed to create dissatisfaction, discontent and desire incessantly invade our psyche. Experts study ways to tap into our innate compulsion for the new or improved, and how to create a must-have desire for something we didn't even know existed before the ad or infomercial. Online and TV shopping enable us to be proud, impulsive owners of widgets and gadgets that may never make it out of the box when it is conveniently deposited at our doorstep.

We're told spending money is good for the economy—until consumers spend more than they have and the economy cascades from a feel-good financial balance to a depressing recession. Obtaining wealth, or the comfortable lifestyle we think wealth can buy, can become a life goal—the sole purpose of our life, in some cases—at the expense of God's best for our life. Too often we believe the lie that we need more money to buy more things to impress more people. Many people fall into the trap of over-consuming, which results in overworking to pay for over-spending. Jesus spoke clearly on these pitfalls.

Read Luke 16:11-14. What master have you chosen to serve?

_____

_____

_____

_____

King Solomon is known as the wisest person who ever lived. When God said that He would give Solomon whatever he wanted, what did Solomon ask for? What did God give him (1 Kings 3:5-14)?

_____

_____

_____

The Lord granted Solomon the wisdom he needed and asked for, but God denied Adam and Eve the wisdom they longingly wanted and craved (Genesis 2:16-17; 3:6-7). What was the difference between the two scenarios?

_____

_____

_____

_____

Solomon describes the value of wisdom in Proverbs 3:

The man who finds wisdom, gains _____ (verse 13).

[Wisdom] is more profitable than _____ and yields better returns than_____ (verse 14).

[Wisdom] is more precious than _____; nothing you desire _____ with her (verse 15).

[Wisdom has] _____ _____ in her right hand; in her left hand are _____ and _____ (verse 16).

[Wisdom's] ways are _____ _____, and all her paths are _____ (verse 17).

[Wisdom] is a _____ ___ _____ to those who embrace her; those who lay hold of her will be _____ (verse 18).

What elements make up wisdom (see 1 Kings 3:9; Proverbs 3:21)?

_____

_____

_____

Do you agree with Solomon that a discerning heart capable of distinguishing right from wrong is more valuable than wealth? Why or why not?

_____

_____

_____

Read Luke 12:29-32. (Although we read this account earlier in Matthew, while discussing appearance, we'll look at Luke's version with an eye on our finances.) Who goes after the things of the world (see verse 30)?

_____

_____

_____

Who knows what we need (see verse 30). What must we do to have our needs met (see verse 31)?

_____

_____

_____

Adam and Eve wanted God's knowledge and wisdom at any cost, and it cost them everything. There's a wealth of wisdom awaiting everyone who seeks the glorious riches of God's kingdom. Ask yourself whether you've bought into the world's pseudo wisdom that more will make you happy, or you are wise in the Lord's ways of achieving wealth that money can't buy. Make sure that what you pursue here on earth is worth the eternal price you might be paying.

Jesus, I hope that, like Solomon, I would choose wisdom and understanding over everything the world offers. Please enter my mind and soul with Your discerning wisdom and help me use my resources for Your glory. Amen.

WHERE'S YOUR TREASURE? Day 3

Dear Lord, in my heart I know You are my most valuable treasure, yet resisting the world's values is so difficult. Guide me in Your value system.

We've all fallen prey to thinking, *If I just had a little bit more* _____ , *then I'd be satisfied.* We could fill in that blank with things like money, clothes, shoes, time or food. These items can satisfy needs, but when they become excessive wants that never satisfy, or we value them more than God, they transcend from necessity to being an idol—something we value more than God. Remember what God said:

> You shall have no other gods before me. You shall not make for yourself an idol in the form of anything in heaven above or on the earth beneath or in the waters below (Exodus 20:3-4).

You can often tell what someone values most by looking at his or her checkbook or credit card statements. Think about your own spending habits. Is there any area of your life in which excessive amounts of money are spent? Have you ever exceeded your credit card limit in order to buy something you wanted but didn't really need? Have you ever spent more than what you've budgeted for something? If you answered yes to any of these questions, briefly explain why you overspent.

_____

_____

_____

Jesus said that we don't need to worry about what we have or don't have; He said we should "seek his kingdom, and these things [what we need] will be given to [us] as well" (Matthew 12:31). Now look at the conclusion of that passage. According to Luke 12:34, Jesus said:

For where your _____ is, there your _____ will be also.

Every aspect of looking at God's best for your life comes back to your motivations, intentions, emotions, thoughts and beliefs. What you treasure most will define your life. Perhaps you've read or heard the story of Sodom and Gomorrah, a city so sinful that God decided to destroy it, but Abraham convinced God to save his nephew Lot and Lot's family. What warning did God give Lot (see Genesis 19:15-17)?

_____

_____

_____

Why do you think Lot hesitated before leaving (see Genesis 19:16)? Why do you think Lot's wife looked back (see Genesis 19:26)?

_____

_____

_____

God was ready and willing to provide everything Lot's wife *needed* for a new life, but by disobeying God and longing for lost "treasures," she not only lost those "treasures," but she also lost her life. According to Psalm 119:14, in what could Lot's wife have rejoiced as if she had "great riches"?

_____

_____

_____

According to Luke 12:33, what happens to your earthly treasures, and what happens to your heavenly treasures?

_____

_____

_____

What exactly is "heavenly" treasure, and how do you get it (see 1 Timothy 6:17-19)?

_____

_____

_____

Maybe you've heard it said that "one person's trash is another person's treasure," but heavenly treasures never lose value. If you were told you only had five minutes to gather up everything of value in your home, what would you take with you?

_____

_____

_____

If those items were your only earthly treasures, how would it affect you (see Luke 12:15)? How would it affect your worth to God?

_____

_____

_____

Our true worth is not based on the accumulation of money or on our possessions; it is determined by our heavenly treasure that we store up by obeying God. No one has ever taken a storage unit, a stock-market portfolio or a U-Haul trailer to heaven! Be generous with your earthly treasures, and never exchange eternal riches for temporary gain.

Dear God, help me hold everything of this world with an open hand. Amen.

Day 4 — FINANCIALLY FIT OR FLAT?

Lord, all I have comes from You, and I'm so grateful. Daily, I want to show my appreciation for Your gifts. Amen.

We're to use heavenly wisdom to make wise earthly financial choices so we can care for our family and our needs with what God provides. We can do this fairly easily if we follow five principles.

Principle 1: Earn it. It only makes sense to have earning money as the first principle, because you have to earn money in order to spend it or allocate it. What do Proverbs 21:25 and 1 Timothy 5:8 have to say about earning a living?

_____

_____

_____

_____

_____

Principle 2: Give it. Read Mark 12:17 and Luke 12:16-21. Giving generously to God should be a natural reaction to whatever provision you have, because God is the One who has provided you with everything you own. The key to wise use of money is seeing how much you can use for God's purposes. If you have money for your wants, but none for God's "wants," that's a lose-lose scenario. Tithing can actually free you from the grip of money. After all, you can't say you truly love God with *all* of your heart if you love money more. God knows what's in your wallet and what's in your heart (see Luke 12:34)!

If you are already tithing, well done! If not, what "wants" or unnecessary expenditures could you eliminate to tithe 10 percent of your income? Where else might you give to the Lord's work and share some of your bounty (see Nehemiah 8:10)?

_____

_____

_____

_____

_____

Principle Three: Save it. Read Proverbs 13:11 and 21:20. Unfortunately, emergencies may happen at any time, and it's always a good idea to have some money put aside to deal with them. Why is saving some of your money a good idea?

_____

_____

_____

_____

Principle 4: Repay it. Read Proverbs 22:7,26-27. We can indulge our wants with a simple swipe of a card and signature, but the bill always arrives and unpaid credit with ensuing interest has sent many into financial crisis. The key to avoiding future debt is practical: don't spend what you don't have. Pay bills, buy necessities, don't buy anything else unless there's money available, and ask God to keep you accountable to this solution. Why is a borrower a slave to the one who does the lending?

_____

_____

_____

Principle 5: Enjoy it. Look up Ecclesiastes 5:18-20. God wants you to enjoy the fruits of your labor with what's left over after practicing the first four principles. Although God's desire is that we enjoy His provision, what is it that brings true joy to our life?

_____

_____

_____

Father, You so richly provide everything I need. Help me to incorporate your money-management principles in my lifestyle. Let my heart always be generous toward You and others. Amen.

Day
5

RICH IN CHRIST?

Jesus, I'm amazed You would invest Your life for me. I pray for a good return on Your investment. Amen.

According to our memory verse, God promises to meet all our needs according to His definition of our needs. From His perspective, a rich spiritual life is more important than a rich portfolio. God wants us freed from the world's wealth and bound to heaven's riches. Sometimes, however, we become so focused on the first part of Philippians 4:19 that we feel it's our right to receive from God, rather than *His* sovereign right to determine what and when He provides. Read Ephesians 1:18-23; 3:16-17. What riches does believing in Christ give us?

_____

_____

_____

Turn to Mark 10:17-23. What two things did Jesus tell the rich young man to do in order to have eternal life, and how did the young man respond?

_____

_____

_____

If the rich man had sold his earthly possessions and given the proceeds to the poor, what would he have gained (see verse 21)?

_____

_____

_____

Read Mark 10:29-30. How did Ruth exemplify what Jesus said?

_____

_____

_____

Read Proverbs 14:31 and Luke 12:16-21. How could a person share his or her wealth, both in regard to money and possessions, with others?

_____

_____

_____

How could a person share his or her spiritual wealth with others?

_____

_____

_____

Look up Proverbs 14:14, John 14:2-3 and Ephesians 2:6-9. What has God promised to those who obey His commands?

_____

_____

_____

God may not ask you to give up all you have to follow Him, but He will ask you to put Him above all you have. You won't be disappointed with the exchange rate. It's an eternal investment that never stops paying dividends.

Jesus, I want to focus on heavenly treasures rather than on earthly treasures.
I love You, Jesus, more than anything this earth could ever offer. Amen.

REFLECTION AND APPLICATION

Father, I want to keep my financial situation in perspective to the bigger picture of my riches in Jesus Christ. Amen.

Have you heard anyone say, "I have enough money, and I don't want any more"? Instead, most of us think that life would be easier, better, happier, less stressful if we had just a little more. But ask a rich person if his or her life is easier, better, happier, less stressful, and he or she will probably tell you no. The amount of money you have doesn't matter; what matters is what you think of money and what you do with what you have. Is God your master, or is money your master?

Money doesn't fill emotional emptiness. Only Jesus can fill that hole permanently and bring satisfaction and peace. If you have Jesus, you have everything you need. As one pastor said, "What I've come to realize is what I have in Christ is far greater than what I don't have in life."

To confirm that you have gained a good perspective on money and what it can and cannot do, complete the following list. Money will buy . . .

A bed but not	<u>rest</u>
Books but not	_____
Food but not	_____
Exercise equipment but not	_____
Clothes but not	_____
A house but not	_____
Medicine but not	_____
Luxuries but not	_____
Amusements but not	_____
Religion but not	_____
A good life but not	_____
A passport to everywhere but not	<u>heaven</u>

How you handle your finances is a good indicator of who, or what, has lordship in your life. What money-management principles do you need to start following or need to improve?

_____

_____

_____

_____

Lord, I'm wealthy and rich in many blessings. Help me remember that only Your riches can truly satisfy and bring joy to my life. Help me remember this truth when my flesh wants to value anything besides You. Amen.

REFLECTION AND APPLICATION

Day 7

Abba, Father, please assist me in applying all I have learned this week. Help me make wise choices in how I earn and spend my money. Teach me Your ways and don't let me be fooled by worldly enticements. Amen.

Don't let a tight budget be an excuse for not eating healthy. Just as tithing and saving is God's best for your life, so is eating nutritiously. Read Isaiah 55:1 from *THE MESSAGE*:

Why do you spend your money on junk food, your hard-earned cash on cotton candy? Listen to me, listen well: Eat only the best, fill yourself with only the finest. Pay attention, come close now, listen carefully to my life-giving, life-nourishing words.

Why we spend our hard-earned money on things like junk food is a question God wants us to consider. Maybe it provides a few moments of comfort or pleasure while we eat it, but after the last bite, we're enveloped in guilt and shame for eating something we shouldn't and wasting money.

Setting a budget for how much to spend on groceries each week and committing to buy only what's on your grocery list can help curtail impulse buying and eating. Unfortunately for us, grocery stores don't help with this discipline. Their marketing goal is to lure and tempt you into impulse purchases.

Take next week's grocery list to the store and observe the following five traps awaiting you. Armed with knowledge, you'll be a wise and prudent shopper.

Trap #1: **Entrance area.** Markets call this the chill zone, designed and decorated to help you visualize fun eating occasions. For example, cartons of soda might be displayed with bags of chips, suggesting a barbecue or beach outing.

Trap #2: **Produce department.** Produce is usually located near the front of the store, because if you shop for such healthy foods first, you're less likely to feel guilty if you indulge in buying unhealthy foods elsewhere. Produce also has the highest profit margin for a grocery store, and a lot of people are less disciplined at the beginning of their shopping trip. Buy produce last and only what you need. (It will get less bruised on top of the cart anyway.)

Trap #3: **Specials.** Located throughout the store are specially marked sale items (these are often highlighted in the store circular). Almost anything specially priced is a good deal, but only if the item is something you need. If you don't need it, don't buy it.

Trap #4: **Strategic placement.** Impulse products such as snacks, candy, cookies and soft drinks are often strategically placed at ends of aisles and at checkout stands. The supermarket is counting on catching your eye or your child's attention and luring you to purchase the products.

Trap #5:   **Buried products.** Popular items are often shelved in the middle of an aisle, so you have to pass other enticing products to get to the one you need.

Describe any other traps you've observed on your shopping trips or any traps that are a hazard to you personally.

_____

_____

_____

_____

Grocery stores are in the business to make money, and they're not watching out for your nutritional health or your finances. If you only put in your cart what's on the grocery list, you can afford to eat healthy. Don't be fooled.

Dear Father, You're amazing! I owe You my life and Your Word tells me You paid my debt in full. I don't always feel worthy of such a sacrifice, but Your love assures me that I am. Amen.

Note

1. Jay Lindsay, "Many Mine Bible for Money Wisdom During Downturn," *The Herald Sun*, August 31, 2010. http://www.heraldsun.com/pages/full_story/push?article-Many+mine+Bible+for+money+wisdom+during+downturn%20&id=5289014.

Group Prayer Requests

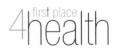

Today's Date: _____

Name	Request

Results

_____

_____

_____

_____

_____

_____

God's best for your daily life

SCRIPTURE MEMORY VERSE

Joshua told the people, "Consecrate yourselves, for tomorrow the LORD will do amazing things among you."

JOSHUA 3:5

Our memory verse this week comes from the Old Testament at an important time in the lives of the Israelites. Moses had just died, and Joshua was the new leader who would take them across the Jordan River and into the Promised Land. They were in anticipation of a holy moment. The Ark of the Covenant would go before them; and, just as He did at the Red Sea, God would part the Jordan for them to cross over on dry land (see Joshua 3:3-4, 14-17). The Israelites were about to participate in an amazing miracle, and Joshua was preparing them for it both physically and spiritually.

Today, we experience God's blessings and miracles on a daily basis, but just as the Israelites needed to be spiritually clean and ready to experience God's presence, so do we. Daily, we need to consecrate ourselves to God and live by the Spirit in every aspect of our daily lives.

DAILY CLEANSING

Day 1

Lord, thank You for always accepting me just the way I am and for giving me the opportunity to go forth washed clean, white as snow. Amen.

In Ruth 3:1-4, Naomi gave Ruth instructions that we might find rather odd today. However, this was part of the normal tradition in the culture of Judah during Bible times. How did Naomi tell Ruth to prepare for this ritual (see verse 3)?

_____

_____

_____

In Joshua 3:5, Joshua told the Israelites to "consecrate yourselves." Moses also told them to consecrate themselves before meeting God at Mount Sinai. Look up Exodus 19:10-11,14-15. What did Joshua and Moses mean?

_____

_____

_____

Moses' and Joshua's instructions to take a bath and wear clean clothes were an outward sign of inward spiritual preparation to worship or serve God. During Bible times, consecration usually also involved a ritualistic animal sacrifice (see Exodus 29:1-3,21), and in the New Testament, the use of "consecrate" refers to this ritual. Read Hebrews 7:26-27; 9:28. What sacrifice was made to fulfill our need to be consecrated?

_____

_____

_____

Jesus' blood sacrificed on the cross for sinners made it possible for Christians to receive a heart and soul cleansing (see Isaiah 1:18). What sacrifices does God ask of us (Psalm 51:16-17)?

_____

_____

_____

Unfortunately, we don't stay clean and contrite—we sin again . . . and again . . . Jesus demonstrated the necessity for daily internal cleansing by outwardly washing the disciples' dirty feet at the Last Supper. Read John

13:1-17. When Peter protested Jesus washing his feet, what did Jesus reply (see verse 10)?

_____

_____

_____

Peter and the disciples were guilty of pride and arrogance (see Luke 22:24), and Jesus gave them a spiritual-cleansing lesson in humility. When He finished, what did Jesus instruct them to do (see John 13:13-17)?

_____

_____

_____

Jesus didn't just mean for the disciples literally to wash people's feet, but He wanted them to follow His humble example of serving others. In what ways do you, or could you, figuratively follow Jesus' instruction "that you should do as I have done for you"?

_____

_____

_____

Read James 5:16. If you stray from your First Place 4 Health program, ask others to pray for you, and then let them know where you got off track. Use Psalm 51:1-12 as a prayer for future daily heart cleansings. What does Psalm 51:13-15 instruct you to do after you're cleansed?

_____

_____

_____

_____

Dear Jesus, I am sorry for disappointing You by sinning. Today, I ask for Your forgiveness and that You would continue to help me overcome my shortcomings. Let me experience the blessings of victory. Amen.

HOLY LIVING

Lord, sometimes I feel so foolish for making mistakes. Thank You for being my Father. I want to be obedient to You and live in Your ways. Amen.

The result of consecration is holiness, a supreme attribute of God. We may think "holy" only refers to God, but He calls every Christian to live a pure and holy daily life. God is holy *all* the time. Look at 1 Peter 1:14-16. What did Peter say about our holiness?

_____

_____

_____

The word "holy" in both Hebrew and Greek means to be set apart for God. Read Leviticus 11:44-45. Why are God's people to be holy?

_____

_____

_____

According to Romans 8:1-9 and 13:8-10, how does the Holy Spirit help us walk in holiness?

_____

_____

_____

The Greek word for "Christian," *christianos*, means "follower of Christ" and is sometimes rendered "little Christ." When we follow the Holy Spirit's guidance, He enables us and empowers us to follow Jesus' example of holiness. Review Romans 8:9-17.

Who should control us (see v. 9)? _____

Who lives in Christians (see vv. 9-10)? _____

What is our obligation (see vv. 12-13)? _____

Whose children are we (see vv. 14-17)? _____

When we sin, why can't we use the excuse "I'm only human"?

_____

_____

_____

Our identity is found in Christ, who is our role model (see 2 Corinthians 3:18). While we will never achieve His perfection in our earthly bodies, perfection is the goal for which we strive. Read Romans 12:1-2. What did the apostle Paul urge believers to do?

_____

_____

_____

As a believer, achieving God's best for your daily life requires aligning your thinking with God's thinking and letting His Spirit lead, guide and empower you. Living holy lives for Christ entails moment-by-moment decisions not to conform to the world's ways but to train your mind—your thought life—to listen to the Holy Spirit's guidance and conform to God's Word and His ways. In the following chart, list some of the world's unholy ways that you should renounce. Then list the way the Holy Spirit can transform your mind as you make the change.

Renouncing the world's ways	Resulting mind transformation
Stop watching R-rated movies	*Removal of sinful images and language*

Jesus, help me to renounce anything distasteful to You. Help me to tune my attention to Your Spirit and receive Your power to retrain my mind. Amen.

Day 3

SET APART

Lord, sometimes it's lonely being the only Christian in a group. Help me stay strong, withstand temptation and always be ready to share what You have done in my life. Amen.

A Christian T-shirt depicts a school of fish swimming together, except for one fish swimming in the opposite direction. As Christians, we sometimes feel like that lone fish: The world's going one way, and we're going another. But that's exactly where God wants us—nonconforming to society's definition of acceptable behavior. While our God is a diverse God, He doesn't condone sinful diversity. Satan's goal is to normalize sin, so we're no longer alarmed when we see it or hear about it. Satan wants our holy antennas to stop going up so that in our complacency, we don't publicly disagree with sinful practices or lifestyles—we don't make waves.

Making holy waves is our job. God wants us swimming upstream against the flow, and that requires standing out and standing up for what we believe. God set us apart for a reason (see Leviticus 20:26). "Set apart" doesn't mean that we remove ourselves from the world; rather, it means that we don't do worldly things and we don't act the way the world acts. We serve our holy God in the way we live our lives each day.

Read John 15:18-20 and John 17:14-17. How might someone react to seeing that you are set apart?

_____

_____

_____

_____

Read 1 Peter 3:8-11. How is a Christian to live a holy life?

_____

_____

_____

_____

How does God feel about those who do evil (see verse 12)?

_____

_____

_____

How do you usually respond when others don't understand or actually challenge your Christian values and beliefs? How should you respond (see 1 Peter 3:14-16)?

_____

_____

_____

What should you do when you're tempted by the world and you forget that you are holy and your life should be holy?

_____

_____

_____

Abba, Father, You see me as holy and consecrated. Transform me, Lord, into a person worthy of the holiness You expect of me. Amen.

YOU'RE A SAINT! Day 4

Dear Father, I love You, and I pray that the Holy Spirit radiates from me at all times. I can't overcome my wayward tendencies without the Holy Spirit's constant guiding in my daily life. Thank You for giving Your Spirit to us. Amen.

First Peter 3:15 tells us to "set apart Christ as Lord" in our hearts, and set apart is how to live a holy life in Christ. "Set apart" is translated from a Greek word, *hagiazo*, which also can be translated as "be holy," "sanctify" or "consecrate." Sanctification, or consecration, occurs when sovereign God sets apart a person, place or thing to accomplish His purpose. It is a progressive development of holiness in character, and God expects consecrated, holy, set-apart Christians to live a moral, ethical, pure life.

What did God sanctify in Genesis 2:3?

_____

_____

_____

Just as God set apart the Sabbath as a holy day, when we became Christians, we were immediately sanctified, set apart and "called to be saints" (Romans 1:7). The process of transforming us into the image of Christ began. According to John 17:17, how did Jesus say we are sanctified?

_____

_____

_____

You might be thinking, *I'm not a saint! There's no way I can live a pure and holy life.* But God's Word says that you are a saint devoted to God for life (see Romans 1:6-7). Now read Psalm 31:23-24. What does God expect of His saints?

_____

_____

_____

Read Psalm 85:8. As saints saved by God's grace, what are we warned not to do?

_____

_____

_____

Turn to 1 Corinthians 6:12. How do Paul's statements counter the claim that because God made food, we should be able to eat anything we want?

_____

_____

_____

Read Psalm 24:4. How could misuse of food lead to sinful or immoral behavior?

_____

_____

_____

_____

How do the following Scriptures advise you to maintain, or regain, clean hands and a pure heart? Follow the example provided.

Scripture	Ways to maintain purity
Job 8:5-7	_Look to God and ask for help._
Ps. 51:9-11	
Ps. 119:9,16	
Prov. 20:11-12	
Phil. 1:9-11	
1 Tim. 1:5	
2 Tim. 2:22	
1 John 1:9	
1 John 3:3	

Those whose sins have been forgiven have "clean hands and a pure heart," but no one is without sin (see Romans 3:23). Never stop asking God for daily cleansing, because "blessed are the pure in heart, for they will see God" (Matthew 5:8).

Holy Lord, I long to see You on that glorious day when we meet face to face in eternity. Until that tomorrow, let me live set apart, sanctified as a witness to Your amazing grace and love for all who put their trust in You. Amen.

Day 5

IT'S A MIRACLE!

Lord, You're an amazing miracle worker. I see Your hand every day in the activities of my life in ways I know could only be You. Make me ready to help others see Your miraculous hand at work in their lives, too. Amen.

The final words in this week's memory verse explain why we need daily cleansing in order to help maintain our sanctity so that we're ready for all God has planned for us: "For tomorrow the Lord will do amazing things among you." Think of it: yesterday's tomorrow is today, and every day God wants to do amazing things in and through you—now that's amazing!

Ruth was infertile during her 10-year marriage to Mahlon (see Ruth 1:4-5). What amazing thing did God do when Ruth married Boaz (see Ruth 4:13-17), and what was God's purpose and plan for this amazing thing (see verse 17)?

_____

_____

_____

_____

In this week's memory verse, we read, "Joshua told the people, 'Consecrate yourselves, for tomorrow the LORD will do amazing things among you.'" Some Bible translations interpret "amazing things" as miracles. In a thesaurus or dictionary, locate synonyms for the word "amazing" and write those below.

_____

_____

_____

_____

The Lord of the Universe has a plan to use you for astounding, remarkable, wonderful, and miraculous things! Are you ready? Are your hands clean and your heart pure? If so, what assurance do you receive from Psalm 25:11-12 that God will reveal when and where He wants to use you?

_____

_____

_____

Read Acts 13:2-12 for an example of how God uses His people who are ready. How did Barnabas and Paul consecrate themselves (and why were they "set apart" (see verse 2)?

_____

_____

_____

What was God's purpose for them (see verse 5)?

_____

_____

_____

What amazing things did the Lord do among them (see verse 12)?

_____

_____

_____

Barnabas and Paul were set apart for the divine purpose of going out into the world as evangelists, and amazing things happened: people accepted Christ as their Savior! God may not be calling you to be an evangelist or missionary, but He does want to do amazing things among the people your life touches. Hearing your story of life before and after Jesus, and observing you living out _God's Best for Your Life_, will be a witness to others.

> _Mighty God, to think that You have a specific purpose and plan for my life is incredible. I don't want to miss it! Help me live the best life I can for You and for Your glory. I'm ready when You are. Amen._

Day
6

REFLECTION AND APPLICATION

Dear Lord, sometimes I find it difficult to think of myself as holy and a saint. But I believe Your Word, and I believe that if I cleanse myself and live my life by obeying Your commands, You will do amazing things in my life. Amen.

This week's memory verse describes the need of the Israelites to cleanse and sanctify themselves in order to participate in a miracle. They followed Joshua's instructions to consecrate themselves and reaped the rewards of their faith. Pastor Rick Warren described this historic event in his book *The Purpose Driven Life*:

> Throughout the Bible we see an important truth illustrated over and over: The Holy Spirit releases his power *the moment* you take a step of faith. When Joshua was faced with an impossible barrier, the floodwaters of the Jordan River receded only *after* the leaders stepped into the rushing current in obedience and faith. Obedience unlocks God's power. God waits for you to act first. Don't wait to feel powerful or confident. Move ahead in your weakness, doing the right thing in spite of your fears and feelings. This is how you cooperate with the Holy Spirit, and it is how your character develops.[1]

You may face what you think are impossible situations in your life or you may think that your goals in First Place 4 Health are unrealistic, but imagine if the Israelites had refused to prepare themselves for the amazing things God wanted to do among them. God wants to do amazing things among the participants of your First Place 4 Health group as well. How can you keep each other accountable in consecrating yourselves for the miracles God plans for each of your lives? List five ideas to share with the group at your next meeting.

1. _____

2. _____

3. _____

4. _____

5. _____

What amazing things do you want to see God do in each area of your life? How can you help each of these miracles take place?

Physically

_____

_____

_____

_____

Mentally

_____

_____

_____

Emotionally

_____

_____

_____

Spiritually

_____

_____

_____

Father, there is no barrier to the amazing things You can do. When I am weak and fear something is impossible, help me to act—to take that first step out in faith to You, knowing that You want to do great things in my life. I'm so very grateful for your love and patience, and I want my everyday life to reflect how I feel about You. Amen.

Day 7

REFLECTION AND APPLICATION

Jesus, I may have a long way to go in approaching purity, but I know it's an achievable goal. With Your encouragement, I'll keep on growing so that every move I make says that "Jesus lives in me." Praise You, Lord.

Sanctification and transformation take time because we each have an inner battle that rages between obeying God and doing good, and yielding to temptations and doing wrong things. Each of us is God's child, but Satan isn't going to surrender without a fight. That's why your daily life must include confession of sins. This will allow God to help you change and grow into Christ's holiness.

In 1 Corinthians 10:13, Paul states, "No temptation has seized you except what is common to man. And God is faithful; he will not let you be tempted beyond what you can bear. But when you are tempted, he will also provide a way out so that you can stand up under it." This passage confirms that God won't give us more than we can handle; but He will strengthen our faith through purifying circumstances. While we're in the heat of the spiritual battle, we may need to physically set ourselves apart from circumstances tempting us to sin.

You've heard the adage "Garbage in, garbage out"? Well, that can apply not only to information but also to circumstances. Think in terms of removing yourself from a situation, or changing the dynamics of a circumstance, in order to prevent "garbage in." For example, if friends insist on viewing movies that are inappropriate for a saintly Christian, excuse yourself. Or if socializing with friends always involves going to lunch, suggest doing something physical, like bowling or tennis. Set yourself apart to be successful in the convictions and commitments you made to God and to yourself.

Today, sit quietly and ask God, "Where do I need to work with You in my sanctification process?" Keep this page open and a pen handy and, as God brings to mind convicting areas in your daily life to change or eliminate, write them below. Consider not just the "big" sins but also small daily sins—going over the speed limit, gossiping, having a critical attitude, and so forth. When you've finished this cleansing time, pray over the list and commit to starting the "clean up" in your daily life, now.

_____

_____

_____

_____

_____

_____

_____

_____

Consider making a banner on your computer or on index cards that reads, "Good in, Good out!" Tape the cards to your TV, computer, refrigerator, steering wheel, phone or any other place that causes you to stumble. While working through your earthly sanctification, it's comforting to know that someday, when you see Jesus face to face, you will be perfect (see Hebrews 10:14)!

> *Dear Lord, I give myself to You wholly and completely. Help me live daily set apart from the world but close to You in my heart. Let Your Holy Spirit sanctify me and filter out the bad, so the good will shine and sparkle. I want my daily life to bring You glory and honor. Amen.*

Note

1. Rick Warren, *The Purpose Driven Life* (Grand Rapids, MI: Zondervan, 2002), pp. 174-175.

Group Prayer Requests

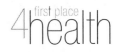

Today's Date: _____

Name	Request

Results

_____

_____

_____

_____

_____

_____

God's best for your service and ministry

SCRIPTURE MEMORY VERSE

*My dear brothers, stand firm. Let nothing move you. Always give yourselves fully
to the work of the Lord, because you know that your labor in the Lord is not in vain.*
1 CORINTHIANS 15:58

Former Major General, Dr. William Cohen, author and founder of the
Institute of Leader Arts, conducts seminars on leadership and management. Cohen often asks his audience if they can think of any organization that has all of these attributes:

- The workers work very hard physically, including weekends,
  with little complaint.
- The workers receive no money and little material compensa-
  tion for their services.
- The work is dangerous and workers are frequently injured on
  the job.
- The work is strictly voluntary.
- The workers usually have very high morale.
- The organization has more workers than can be employed.
- The workers are highly motivated to achieve the organiza-
  tion's goals.

Cohen's audience is frequently stumped, thinking there is no organization like this on earth. But Cohen tells them he knows of one: a
high school football team.[1]

As Christians, we know of another: the church! We believers were saved to serve. Finding God's best for your service and ministry is your life's purpose.

Day 1
A NEW BODY IN HEAVEN

Lord, I look forward to the day when I will embrace a new, glorious body in heaven. But while I'm still in my earthly body, help me learn to care for it properly, so I'm able to do the work You set before me. Amen.

The significance of today's memory verse is best appreciated in context. Look up 1 Corinthians 15:58 in your Bible. You'll notice that the first word of the verse is "therefore," indicating a transition or link from a previous thought. Let's investigate the passage prior to verse 58, beginning at verse 35. The heading above this passage in your Bible might read "The Resurrection Body." How does Paul contrast our earthly body with our eternal heavenly body (see verses 40,42-44)?

Earthly body	Heavenly body

Contrast "the first man Adam," with "the last Adam," Jesus (verses 45-48).

Adam's body	Jesus' body

While our earthly body resembles Adam's, our heavenly body will resemble Christ (see verse 49). What do you think about your body not going to heaven with you?

_____

_____

_____

_____

What victory is proclaimed in verses 54-57?

_____

_____

_____

_____

When most bees sting, a stinger is left embedded in our flesh, and such bees, robbed of their sting, die. Similarly, death lost its stinger at the cross, and Satan was robbed of terrorizing us with it ever again. According to 1 Corinthians 15:56, "the law" calls us to accountability by tugging at our conscience and convicting us of sins. The joy of knowing we have a forgiving God, who welcomes forgiven sinners into eternity through victory in Jesus (see verse 57), segues into verse 58. "Therefore," knowing that as a saved Christian your faith is not in vain, what does verse 58 exhort you to do personally?

_____

_____

_____

_____

What is your plan for implementing the challenge of verse 58?

_____

_____

_____

_____

Close today by reading Philippians 3:17–4:1 and mediating on the promise of your glorious heavenly body.

> *Dear Jesus, thank You for Your sacrifice on the cross. Thank You for taking away the sting of death and promising me a glorious spiritual body. Amen.*

Day 2 — STANDING FIRM

Lord, please help me to be strong and to resist anything unhealthy. I know that through Your strength, I will overcome my weaknesses. Amen.

Spiritual warfare usually takes on a physical form in our life. Satan doesn't want us doing the Lord's work, and he will continue to attack us, tempting us to disobey God. Fortunately, with wisdom and discernment, we can recognize Satan's interference in our lives, and we can stand firm in our faith and continue to obey God. Because of the truth of the resurrection, we can face overwhelming or difficult circumstances with hope and steadfastness. How does 1 John 4:4 provide courage to withstand Satan's attempts at distracting you from the work of the Lord?

_____

_____

_____

_____

In Week Three, you studied putting on the armor of God in Ephesians 6:10-18. Reread those verses today. Why do verses 11,13-14 tell you to put on the *full* armor of God?

So that you can take your _____ against the _____ _____.

So that when the day of evil comes, you may be able to _____ _____ _____ and after you have done everything to _____. _____ _____ .

Regardless of how you answered the previous question as to who or what tried to "move you," people are not the source of the assault. Who uses people and circumstances to shake us (see verse 12)?

For our struggle is not against _____ and _____, but against the _____, against the _____ against the _____ of this _____ _____ and against the spiritual forces of _____ in the heavenly realms.

How does knowing Satan's tactics, help refocus and redirect your energy from combating difficult people to fighting Satan instead?

_____

_____

_____

With Christ you are invincible and unmovable. No matter how much Satan tries to huff and puff with suffering, troubles, discouragement and despair, you can stay spiritually strong and not be shaken. In 2 Chronicles 20, Jehoshaphat found himself and all of the Israelites completely surrounded by enemy armies. So he and the people prayed to God for help, and God gave them an answer. Read verses 14-17. What did God advise the people to do? How did He comfort them in this time of need?

_____

_____

_____

Read Matthew 10:22 and 24:12-13. What do we gain by standing firm?

_____

_____

_____

Lord, there are times when I feel surrounded by enemies. Holy Spirit, make me strong to stand firm against the enemy's attempts to weaken my resolve. Amen.

<table>
<tr><td>Day
3</td></tr>
</table>

Day 3 — THE OPPORTUNITY TO SERVE

Dear Father, it's hard for me to imagine You using fallible me to do Your infallible work. Help me understand how I am to do Your will. Amen.

When we become Christians by faith, we also become God's servants. When you're standing firm in the Lord and your faith cannot be shaken, you're ready to seek opportunities to give yourself "fully to the work of the Lord." The Lord's work is actually an *opportunity* not an *obligation* (see Galatians 5:13). Look up the following verses in Ruth and examples of the opportunities that Naomi, Ruth and Boaz found to serve each other.

Scripture	Examples of opportunites
Ruth 1:16-17	
Ruth 2:8-9	
Ruth 3:1-4	

Read 1 Peter 2:9 and Revelation 5:9-10. How are Christians described?

_____

_____

_____

Last week you learned you were a saint, and now you are a "priest" in the "royal priesthood"! In *The Purpose Driven Life*, Pastor Rick Warren explains the concept of every Christian being in a priesthood of servants:

> When most people hear "ministry," they think of pastors, priests, and professional clergy, but God says every member of His family is a minister. In the Bible, the words *servant* and *minister* are synonyms, as are *service* and *ministry*. If you are a Christian, you are a minister and when you're serving, you're ministering.[2]

Ministry, "the work of the Lord," occurs every time you help or serve in the name of Jesus—even giving a cup of cold water to someone who is thirsty (see Mark 9:41). You may be thinking, *I have a job. I have a family. How could I do full-time work for the Lord?* Read Matthew 25:37-40 and 1 Peter 4:9-10. What does the Lord's work actually involve?

_____

_____

_____

God doesn't want dutiful serving. Read Romans 12:10-11, Romans 14:19 and Ephesians 6:7. What kind of servant does God want?

_____

_____

_____

Who is our example of servant ministry (see Mark 10:45; Philippians 2:7)?

_____

_____

_____

In what practical ways can you serve people you know? In what practical ways can you serve people you don't know?

_____

_____

_____

Serving God today is a dress rehearsal for an eternity of serving Him; and those whom we serve on earth in His name have an opportunity to be serving right beside us in heaven (see Revelation 7:14-15; 22:3).

Jesus, You came to earth to humbly show us how to serve and love our fellow man. Help me take my eyes off myself and my needs, and help me look for opportunities to fulfill the needs of others in Your name. Amen.

A LABOR OF LOVE

*Dear Lord, Help me to recognize that any work I do for You is never in vain.
Give me a right attitude of a love that never gives up. Amen.*

It's been said that the reason some people don't recognize opportunity is because it usually comes disguised as hard work! Kingdom work doesn't always have tangible results or rewards, and it is easy to lose hope of ever making a difference. Your resolve to remain steadfast can slip away, and you may consider only looking out for yourself and letting someone else serve God. Anticipating these concerns, Paul added the last phrase to our memory verse: "You know that Your labor in the Lord is not in vain." No one knew better than Paul the arduousness of ministry work.

Read 2 Corinthians 6:4-10, and then note Paul's positive attitude about his hardships in verses 9-10:

Dying, and yet we _____ _____;

beaten, and yet _____ _____;

sorrowful, yet _____ _____;

poor, yet _____ _____ _____;

having nothing, and yet _____ _____;

Now read 2 Corinthians 4:7-9 and fill in the following:

But we have this treasure in jars of clay to show that this all-surpassing power is from God and not from us. We are hard pressed on every side, but _____ _____; perplexed, but _____ _____ _____ ; persecuted, but _____ _____; struck down, but _____ _____.

In addition to being a traveling evangelist, Paul had a career as a tent-maker (see Acts 18:3), yet he found time to write encouraging and discipling letters to the new Christian churches. He championed the message that even though spreading the Gospel involves hard work, we should never give up because our efforts count. Paul made a difference for the Kingdom, and when faced with persecution and rejection, he pressed on toward the goal of someday being with Christ and taking as many people with him as he could (see Philippians 3:14). What other words did Paul use in the following verses to describe "not in vain"?

2 Corinthians 4:1

_____
_____
_____

Philippians 2:14-16

_____
_____
_____

1 Thessalonians 2:1

_____
_____
_____

1 Thessalonians 3:5

_____
_____
_____

Occasionally, we all fear our labor might be in vain. Where do you feel like that right now? Is your work at weight loss and exercise producing anticipated results?

_____
_____
_____
_____

What if Paul had said that the Lord's work was too tough and had quit? We wouldn't have the wisdom and teachings of almost half the New Testament! Paul never knew the future value of his labor of love in writing letters to the churches. In the same way, God sees the work you're doing and, while you may not see desired results, He wants you to keep on persevering. In the following table, look up the Scripture in the left-hand column and list the ways that we can be encouraged to persevere.

Scripture	I'm encouraged to persevere because . . .
Deut. 2:7	
Rom. 16:12-13	
1 Thess. 1:3	
Heb. 6:10	
Rev. 14:13	

We never know how the Lord will use us in His work force, so we must stay trained, equipped and ready for wherever and whenever He calls. Someday, workers laboring out of love for God and others will hear the words, "Well done, good and faithful servant! You have been faithful with a few things; I will put you in charge of many things. Come and share your master's happiness!" (Matthew 25:21).

Thank You, Lord, for loving me. Help me put my life's tasks in perspective, so I'll focus more on Your work and making it a part of my lifestyle. Amen.

Day 5 — THE WORKERS OF THE LORD

Precious Lord, I will learn and share with others how You satisfy hunger and thirst forever. Let me be a faithful worker in your harvest field. Amen.

God's harvest field is the world—everywhere and everyone who needs to hear the good news. God assigns believers the task of planting or watering the seed of faith in unbelievers, no matter how hard or dry the heart soil.

Sometimes our job is to toil at digging, planting and watering. Other times, our task is easier—we harvest someone else's hard work. God will do the even harder work of making the tiny seed grow and flower into faith. In the chart below, describe the opportunity to serve for each worker.

Worker of the Lord	Description of opportunity to serve
Planters of the seed (see 1 Cor. 3:6-8)	
Waterers of the seed of faith (1 Cor. 3:6-8)	
Growers cultivating and nourishing the seed (see Rom. 15:1-8)	
Harvesters reaping a crop for eternal life (see John 4:35-38)	

Read John 4:1-42. What did Jesus ask of the woman, and why did the woman find the request odd (see verses 7,9)?

How did Jesus use a universal need as an opportunity to share the gospel (see verses 10-26)?

What was the reaction of the disciples, and what was the outcome of the new believer sharing her good news (see verses 27,39-42)?

While discussing water, a necessity of life, a woman accepted Jesus as the Messiah: a successful fulfillment of the work His Father had sent Him to do, and the job for which He tried to train His workers. But what were His workers, the disciples, focused on (see verses 31-33)?

_____

_____

_____

How did Jesus respond to the disciples' concern with earthly food (see verse 34)?

_____

_____

_____

You don't have to be a missionary or be on a church staff to work for God. He'll use you right where you are by presenting opportunities to serve Him in your daily life. Your job may be as simple as opening a conversation by asking, "Will you give me a drink?" Or boldly sharing, "Come, see a man who told me everything I ever did." Just as the Lord "loves a cheerful giver" (2 Corinthians 9:7), so He values a cheerful worker. What will you gain for your hard work? Read King Solomon's answer in Ecclesiastes 3:9-14, and then describe the satisfaction you find in your toil.

_____

_____

_____

_____

In light of an eternity spent with our heavenly employer, Jesus Christ, work for the Lord is never meaningless or too hard.

Dear God, I truly want to be part of Your workforce. Provide me words and opportunities to share my testimony, and I'll tell of the mighty wonders I've seen You do in my life. Amen.

REFLECTION AND APPLICATION

*Heavenly Father, there are days when I feel like I am losing ground.
Help me to stand firm when my determination and resolve falter. Amen.*

This week, we again saw the importance of prayerfully clothing ourselves in the armor of God. Have you been prayerfully putting on the *full* armor of God daily? If so, have you noticed any difference in how your day goes? If not, why not?

_____

_____

_____

Understanding the significance of the Roman soldier putting on each piece of armor in a particular order should help solidify this Scripture passage in your mind. Read Ephesians 6:10-18. In the picture of the Roman soldier below, write in each piece of armor and its spiritual analogy.

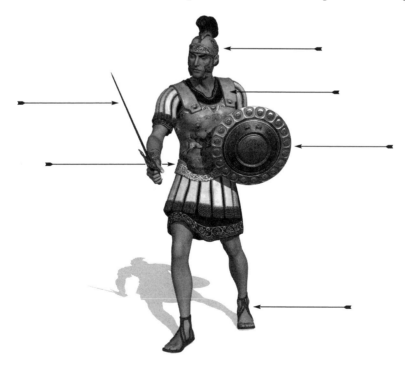

Note the order in which each of these pieces of equipment is listed. The following demonstrates the importance of putting on armor in the correct order:

Roman equipment	Spiritual analogy
Belt of Truth (v. 14): Put on first to tighten loose robe; held sheath for sword and breastplate attached to it	Truth central to Christianity
Breastplate of Righteousness (v. 14): Protected heart and lungs	Pure heart and emotion
Shoes of the Gospel of Peace (v. 14): Studs or nails on soles for a firm footing; no slipping or sliding; soldier could hold his ground on an incline; protection from sharpened sticks implanted in the ground	Prevent backsliding; avoid slipping into temptation; ready to share the gospel; move forward spiritually
Shield of Faith (v. 16): Wood with protective medal coating; repel flaming arrows that might lodge in it	Faith protects against Satan's lies
Helmet of Salvation (v. 17): Made of leather embedded with pieces of metal; designed to withstand a crushing blow to the head	Guard mind and thoughts; remember you are saved
Sword of the Spirit (v. 17): Our only offensive weapon	Use the Word of God

The Roman soldier didn't go to battle alone, and neither can you. We need to stand side by side with other believers, our shields of faith linked together, and demonstrate God's victory in every painful, confusing, and challenging situation.

> *Lord, I will put on the belt of truth, the breastplate of righteousness and the shoes of the gospel of peace. I will lift up the shield of faith to fend off the darts of the evil one and put on the helmet of salvation to protect my mind. I will defend myself with the sword of the Spirit, the Word of God. Amen.*

REFLECTION AND APPLICATION

Dear Lord, help me apply all I've studied this week. I want to be used by You to plant, water, grow and harvest into spiritual fruit for Your kingdom. Amen.

Read and meditate on Ephesians 2:8-11. Think back over the past seven days and recall some of the people whom you have emailed or texted, or talked with by phone or in person. Consider how many opportunities you might have had to serve the Lord by offering your hope, encouragement, love, witness or testimony to these individuals. Don't beat yourself up over missed opportunities, but simply pray and reflect on how you could do things differently. Now, as you go through this next week, keep a list of the people with whom you communicate—those whom you have the opportunity to serve—and note whether you were a planter, waterer, grower or harvester.

Person	Planter	Waterer	Grower	Harvester

Keep a chart like this until working for the Lord becomes a habit. You will be ready to seize opportunities to tell your world—the fertile ground where God planted you.

Jesus, open my eyes to see the work You have set before me and give me a heart ready to make whatever life changes the work might require. Amen.

Notes

1. William A. Cohen, *The Art of the Leader* (Englewood Cliff, NJ: Prentice Hall, 1990), p. 99.
2. Rick Warren, *The Purpose Driven Life: What on Earth Am I Here For?* (Grand Rapids, MI: Zondervan, 2002), pp. 228-29.

Group Prayer Requests

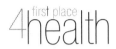

Today's Date: _____

Name	Request

Results

_____

_____

_____

_____

_____

_____

God's best for your future

SCRIPTURE MEMORY VERSE
You prepare a table before me in the presence of my enemies. You anoint my head with oil, my cup overflows. Surely goodness and love will follow me all the days of my life, and I will dwell in the house of the LORD forever.
PSALM 23:5-6

If you ever attended Sunday School as a child, you may have memorized this well-known psalm of King David, which pictures God as a shepherd watching over and caring for His people, the sheep. We usually don't think of ourselves as sheep, but God often refers to His people as sheep, and He is the Good Shepherd who knows each one of us by name and worries if even one goes astray. Perhaps that's why this psalm has spanned the ages as one of the most universally known and repeated passages in Scripture. Even nonbelievers can sometimes be heard reciting it. There is an innate awareness that at the end of the day—the end of our earthly life—God opens the gate to the eternal sheepfold and welcomes in all who call Him Lord.

THE GOOD SHEPHERD
Day 1

Lord, You are my Shepherd. Help me be content with the pastures You provide and to overcome fears I have about the future. Amen.

The Bible mentions sheep, literally and figuratively, more than 500 times. Sheep are "harassed and helpless" (Matthew 9:36), vulnerable to wild animals and prone to go astray, just like people without God. A shepherd's job is to care for and protect his sheep. In both the Old and New Testament, sheep metaphorically represent humans. The shepherd symbolizes (1) human leaders who care for God's flock, (2) God, who accepts responsibility to care for and protect the believer, and (3) Jesus Christ, who as the Good Shepherd gave His life for His sheep. In the following table, list how the Bible describes each of the following shepherd rulers:

Ruler	Scripture	Description
David	2 Sam. 5:1-2	
	Ps. 78:70-72	
God	Gen. 48:15	
	Isa. 40:10-11	
	Jer. 31:10	
	Ezek. 34:11-16	
Jesus	Mic. 5:4-5	
	John 10:1-18	

Read Ezekiel 34:1-10. What are the signs of a shepherd who is not leading his or her flock in the way that God intends (see verses 1-4)?

_____

_____

_____

_____

What happens to a flock with this type of shepherd (see verses 5-6)?

_____

_____

_____

_____

How does God deal with these shepherds (see verses 7-10)?

_____

_____

_____

According to Psalm 95:6-8 and Psalm 100:1-5, how are we—the sheep—to respond to our Good Shepherd, the Lord?

_____

_____

_____

Read 1 Peter 5:1-4, which describes Christian shepherds. How did Naomi shepherd Ruth (see Ruth 3:1-4)?

_____

_____

_____

How did God reward Naomi (see Ruth 4:14-17)?

_____

_____

_____

Who has God put in your "flock" to watch over, encourage and care for; and how will you be a good shepherd to *your* "sheep"?

_____

_____

_____

_____

My Good Shepherd, I feel safe, knowing that I am under Your loving care. Help me not to stray from your ways, and guide me to be a good shepherd to all You entrust to my care. Amen.

BLESSED TO BE A BLESSING

*Lord, You have prepared for me a table of blessings, and You have secured
my safety from the enemy. Thank You. Amen.*

The first half of verse 5 of this week's memory verse, "You prepare a table
before me in the presence of my enemies," may seem a bit unclear, but the
records of ancient history provide a window into David's thoughts when
he wrote this verse. Near Eastern hospitality guaranteed food and security for guests, as J. H. Jowett explains, "All the hallowed sanctions of hospitality gather around him [the guest] for his defense. He is taken into the
tent, food is placed before him, while his evaded pursuers stand frown-
ingly at the door."[1] In the example of the shepherd with his sheep, each
spring, the shepherd dug out and burned poisonous plants that were fa-
tal to the sheep if eaten. By burning these plants—enemies to the sheep—
he made the pastures safe for the sheep to graze. In a sense, the shepherd
prepared a table for the sheep and destroyed their enemy.

How has your Good Shepherd prepared a table for you? With what nour-
ishment have you been provided?

_____

_____

_____

What blessings has God put on the table (see Ephesians 1:3; 2:18; Hebrews 13:5)?

_____

_____

_____

How has God secured your safety from your enemy (see Colossians 1:13)?

_____

_____

_____

Describe a time when you have been in a perilous situation. How did the Shepherd protect you?

How can you help protect the First Place 4 Health flock of which you are a part?

How can you help protect your personal flock?

My Good Shepherd, thank You for the generous gifts You provide for me at Your table. Thank You, too, for Your protection. I don't know what I'd do without You. Help me to follow Your example. Amen.

YOU ARE ANOINTED

Day 3

Lord, it's soothing just thinking about You hovering over my head so close that You see the hurts and are ready to pour over me Your calming, refreshing balm. I want to come to You to feel refreshed. Amen.

Anointing an honored guest's head with oil at a banquet table was another ancient Near Eastern custom. Ceremonious anointing also denoted a king, priesthood and consecration (or sanctification). What is the significance of anointing in the following Scriptures?

Scripture	Use of anointing oil
Exod. 30:30-32	
Exod. 40:9	
Ps. 45:7	
Eccles. 9:7-8	
Luke 7:44-47	

Last week, you learned that you're part of the royal priesthood of Christ, and God anoints you both as a priest and a saint. Shepherds performed another type of anointing. As each sheep came through the doorway of the sheepfold at night, the shepherd examined the sheep's head and applied soothing, healing oil to any cuts and abrasions the sheep may have incurred from stones, briars and thorns. Shepherds also put oil on sheep to repel bugs that could be very annoying and possibly infect the animals.

Sometimes you may feel like a wounded sheep in need of healing anointing, as hidden hurts continue to give you pain. What hidden hurts, what disappointments, continue to give you pain?

According the following verses, what "soothing oils" does God provide?

Scripture	Soothing oil
Ps. 28:8-9	
Isa. 40:11	
Mic. 5:4-5	
1 Pet. 2:24	

Your Great Good Shepherd is concerned about your personal healing and protection. While the Good Shepherd looks after *all* His flock, in His sovereignty, He knows *your* daily struggles. When you pass through the heavenly gate and meet your Good Shepherd, He'll know your name and you will recognize His voice (see John 10:3-4,7). Read Psalm 25:1-2. Where should your trust and hope be? Why?

_____

_____

_____

God wants to heal you and protect you and keep you as His own.

Good Shepherd, with the millions of sheep You have in Your fold, You know my name! I will follow You, for I trust You to heal me and protect me. Amen.

AN OVERFLOWING CUP

Day 4

Jesus, I know that You want to give me more than I could ever imagine. Help me have a surrendered heart ready and willing to do Your will. Amen.

A young scholar traveled a great distance to study at the feet of a revered sage. The young man tried to impress the master with how much he knew and how wise he was. Instead of asking questions, the student carried on about his beliefs and philosophies. The master listened quietly for a long while. Finally, the student stopped talking and the master asked if he would like some tea. "Yes," the young man replied. The old man began pouring the tea into his visitor's cup, but he didn't stop when the cup was full. He continued pouring as the tea overflowed into the saucer, onto the tabletop and onto the floor.

"Stop!" the young man cried, "The cup is full. Can't you see? It can hold no more."

"It's true," the wise one said. "We cannot put more into an already full cup. And you are like that cup. Until you empty yourself of yourself, your fullness will prevent you from learning."

Psalm 23:5 assures us that God wants to shower us with an overflowing abundance of blessings, but first we must empty ourselves of self. How do we sometimes resemble the young scholar when we come before God?

_____

_____

_____

The literal meaning of "cup" in verse 5 is, of course, a vessel used to hold liquid. In Near East culture, a host at a banquet or meal never lets the cup of an honored guest go empty and continues to refill it, encouraging the guest to stay. Scripture also often uses "cup" metaphorically; for example, "cup" in verse 5 is, metaphorically, life. Read Isaiah 51:17-22. What does the "cup" represent in this passage?

_____

_____

_____

Now turn to Matthew 26:27-28. What does the "cup" represent?

_____

_____

_____

Symbolically, God's cup in Scripture referred to a number of different things, including His wrath, salvation, and Jesus and His covenant with us. When we accept Jesus as our personal Savior, we are immediately filled with the Holy Spirit, and our cup of life overflows with blessings. Read Romans 15:13. With what else should your cup be filled?

_____

_____

_____

Earlier in this study, you read in Romans 12:1 about surrendering your life to Christ and devoting your life to serving Him. When you do this, you'll receive God's best for your future, and He will provide more than you could possibly expect. In the cup below, write the blessings you've seen overflow from your salvation and service.

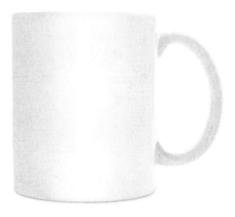

When you experience cravings or tempting desires for food and things you shouldn't have or don't need, return to this overflowing cup of blessings. Imagine *never* being in want for anything—never hungering or thirsting ever again—because the richness of God's love and blessing are more than enough for you. Reach for "the spring of living water" that fills your cup over the brim and satisfies like nothing on earth ever will.

Savior, You filled my cup with blessings to enjoy on earth and my salvation for tomorrow. Help me to share from my overflowing cup of blessings.

A SECURE FUTURE   Day 5
Lord, help me find my security in You and not the world. Amen.

Gilbert Brenken once said, "Other men see only a hopeless end, but the Christian rejoices in an endless hope."[2] There isn't a more beautiful hope-filled promise than "Surely your goodness and unfailing love will pursue me all the days of my life, and I will live in the house of the LORD forever" (Psalm 23:6, *NLT*). It doesn't get much better than that, does it!

David knew prophecies about the coming Messiah, but he didn't have the revelation of an eternal life with Jesus that we have today. David couldn't look into the future and probably couldn't imagine the Easter resurrection to come. But David knew God well enough to know that his future was secure with the Lord, so he began Psalm 23:6 with "surely." What a man of faith!

Read John 11:25-26. What did Jesus mean by His description of Himself?

_____

_____

_____

David went on to say that he would have God's "goodness and love." This sounds wonderful, but David well knew that we would have trials and troubles during our time on earth. So how could we have God's goodness and mercy all the time if we sometimes have bad times? The point is that it is God's goodness that sees us through our hard times. It's His love that gives us strength. Read Psalm 23:4. Why do we not need to be afraid or feel alone, especially during bad times?

_____

_____

_____

David often referred to God as a "refuge." Look up "refuge" in a dictionary. What does this term mean?

_____

_____

_____

Read Psalm 91. How is God our refuge?

_____

_____

_____

Why is God our refuge (see verse 14)?

_____

_____

_____

Since we have God's goodness, why do we need His mercy?

_____

_____

_____

Read Philippians 1:20. Where is our real home?

_____

_____

_____

Father, there is a peace that fills my soul when I consider my future with You,
both here on earth and in heaven. Help me live on earth with heaven in view.

REFLECTION AND APPLICATION

Day 6

My Good Shepherd, I want to know You deeply and completely. I pray
for a relationship with You that surpasses all others in my life. Amen.

There is a story of an old and young man on the same platform before an audience of people. They were participating in a program and each man's part was to repeat from memory the words of the 23rd Psalm. The young man, trained in the best speech and drama techniques, spoke in the language of an ancient silver-tongued orator: "The Lord is my Shepherd . . ."

When he finished, the audience clapped and cheered, asking him for an encore so they might hear again his wonderful voice.

Then the old gentleman, leaning heavily on his cane, stepped to the front of the same platform and in a feeble, shaking voice, repeated the same words—"The Lord is my Shepherd . . ." But when he finished, the listeners were silent and seemed to be praying.

In the profound silence, the young man stood and said, "Friends, I wish to make an explanation. You asked me to come back and repeat the psalm, but you remained silent when my friend was finished. The difference? I shall tell you. I know the psalm, but he knows the Shepherd!" As you reflect back on the study you did this week, ask yourself the following questions and record your answers below.

I know *about* the Shepherd, but do I really *know* the Shepherd?

_____

_____

_____

Has the Shepherd's goodness taken root in me so I'm becoming like Him?

_____

_____

_____

Do I show mercy to others, like God shows to me?

_____

_____

_____

Do I love others as Christ loves me?

_____

_____

_____

This week, make plans to invite someone who doesn't know the Good Shepherd over to your home for a cup of coffee or tea. Share with your guest the story of who fills your cup and your soul to overflowing.

Loving God, I want to sit at Your table and I want to dwell in Your house. Let Your light shine through me and what I can do for You. Amen.

REFLECTION AND APPLICATION

Lord, You are my dwelling place, my refuge and my strength. I couldn't live my life without You. Thank You for making Your home in my heart. Amen.

Robert Boyd Munger, in his little book *My Heart, Christ's Home*, provides a visual of Jesus making His home in his heart, room-by-room. As he tours the rooms of his heart, he realizes that each room needs something cleaned out or needs to be redecorated with something better or more Christlike. As you reflect on this study, look at the rooms in your own heart. Examine each of your rooms, and then tell what you need to clean out of each one and what you would use to redecorate the space with.

Room	Clean out	Use for redecoration
Living Room (where you meet with Jesus daily)		
Dining Room (appetites)		
Library (your mind)		
Workroom (talents and skills)		
Kitchen (nourishment)		
Yard (exercise, physical activity)		
Basement or attic (hidden hurts)		
Closet (hidden sins)		

Thank You, God, for taking up residence in my heart. I'm committed to making the changes revealed to me through this study. Thank You for Your love and strength and mercy. Thank You for being my Father. Amen.

Notes

1. J. H. Jowett, quoted in William MacDonald, *Believer's Bible Commentary* (Nashville, TN: Thomas Nelson Publishers, 1990), p. 581.
2. Gilbert Brenken, quoted in Chris Tiegreen, *The One Year Walk with God Devotional* (Wheaton, IL: Tyndale House Publishers, 2004), April 30.

Group Prayer Requests

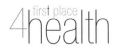

Today's Date: _____

Name	Request

Results

_____

_____

_____

_____

_____

time to celebrate!

To help shape your brief victory celebration testimony, work through the following questions in your prayer journal:

Day One: List some of the benefits you have gained by allowing the Lord to transform your life through this 12-week First Place 4 Health session. Be sure to list benefits you have received in the physical, mental, emotional and spiritual realms of your being.

Day Two: In what ways have you most significantly changed *mentally*? Have you seen a shift in the ways you think about yourself, food, your relationships or God? How has Scripture memory been a part of these shifts?

Day Three: In what ways have you most significantly changed *emotionally*? Have you begun to identify how your feelings influence your relationship to food and exercise? What are you doing to stay aware of your emotions, both positive and negative?

Day Four: In what ways have you most significantly changed *spiritually*? How has your relationship with God deepened? How has drawing closer to Him made a difference in the other three areas of your life?

Day Five: In what ways have you most significantly changed *physically*? Have you met or exceeded your weight/measurement goals? How has your health improved the past 12 weeks?

Day Six: Was there one person in your First Place 4 Health group who was particularly encouraging to you? How did their kindness make a difference in your First Place 4 Health journey?

Day Seven: Summarize the previous six questions into a one-page testimony, or "faith story," to share at your group's victory celebration.

May our gracious Lord bless and keep you as you continue to keep Him first in all things!

God's Best for Your Life
leader discussion guide

For in-depth information, guidance and helpful tips about leading a successful First Place 4 Health group, study the *First Place 4 Health Leader's Guide*. In it, you will find valuable answers to most of your questions, as well as personal insights from many First Place 4 Health group leaders.

For the group meetings in this session, be sure to read and consider each week's discussion topics several days before the meeting—some questions and activities require supplies and/or planning to complete. Also, if you are leading a large group, plan to break into smaller groups for discussion and then come together as a large group to share your answers and responses. Make sure to appoint a capable leader for each small group so that discussions stay focused and on track (and be sure each group records their answers!).

week one: welcome to *God's best for your life*

During this first week, welcome the members to your group, provide a brief overview of the First Place 4 Health program, explain what is expected of the participants at each of the weekly meetings, and collect the Member Surveys. (See the *First Place 4 Health Leader's Guide* for a detailed outline of how to conduct the first week's meeting.)

week two: God's best for your physical life

Discuss items the participants have made from scratch. Then lead a discussion of how God feels about His creation and how His love for us should influence the way we take care of our bodies. Highlight the fact that each and every person is unique—"fearfully and wonderfully made"—and that the body of each believer "is a temple of the Holy Spirit."

On Day Two, participants considered God's best for fueling their unique body with food. Ask them what they learned from the example of the bad choices made by Adam and Eve and by Elimelech and Naomi.

Ensure that the group understands John 6:35 and what Jesus meant by saying He is the bread of life. Discuss our need to feed more on spiritual bread (the Bible) than on physical bread. This would be a good time to talk about physical cravings being a symptom of spiritual cravings.

On Day Three, the focus was on getting healthy and getting enough sleep. Everyone might have a different definition of "healthy," so ask what living a healthy lifestyle signifies to each person.

On Day Four, participants were encouraged to get and stay fit physically, so start off with a discussion of how the group answered the first question (their opinion of exercise in general).

For Day Five, emphasize that everything we do affects our family, not just ourselves. Ask how participants are customizing and applying their First Place 4 Health program for their family.

week three: God's best for your spiritual life

Ask for answers to the significance of Ruth accepting Naomi's God, the one and only true God. Make sure the group understands that Ruth's conversion resulted from observing the godly life of Naomi for the previous 10 years, even while Naomi lived in a pagan land.

Read Acts 2:38 aloud. If anyone accepted Christ the first week, encourage him or her to consider baptism as the next step. Discuss how the fruit of the Spirit listed in Galatians 5:22-23 are reflected in our physical life, from the inside out.

Day Two included a discussion of the armor of God and preparing for battle with the enemy, Satan. Review the spiritual application and the protection of each piece of the armor of God.

Have someone read Psalm 119:11. Point out that the sword of the Spirit—Scripture—is our only offensive weapon. Ask for testimonies of anyone who has experienced the power of Scripture in his or her life.

On a whiteboard make three columns with the headings: "Repent," "Remorse" and "Regret." Have the group give synonyms for each word. Lead a discussion of how remorse and regret are *feeling* sorry about doing something, but the sin will reoccur without repentance.

Read Psalm 63:3-5. Ask participants to share their experience of achieving the same sense of satisfaction from praising God as from eating a favorite food. In closing your time together, sing a joyful praise song.

week four: God's best for your circumstances

On a whiteboard, list the group's answers for "Naomi's and Ruth's Circumstances" and "God's Purpose and Plan." Have someone read aloud Psalm 42:5. Ask what motivated David and Paul to endure tough circumstances and what can help us do the same. Also ask what Paul was doing during his time of hardships and why he could still give thanks.

From Day Four, discuss the witness of the biblical characters. Focus on Ruth observing Naomi's witness of faith while living in Moab, resulting in Ruth accepting Naomi's God, and their time together in Bethlehem.

The story of the paralyzed man in Mark 2:1-12 probably is a familiar one to most Christians. Ask if anyone had ever considered the witness of the four friends rather than focusing on Jesus' healing of the paralytic. Invite personal testimonies of someone doing something similar for them, and the witness it was for friends and family.

Ask volunteers to read Psalm 100 and 1 Thessalonians 5:16-18. Discuss how personalizing these verses could help when God seems distant.

The Day Six study put circumstances into perspective. Discuss looking at each circumstance through God's eyes—as an opportunity to effect change or be satisfied—in any case as an opportunity to serve Him.

As a group, personalize and pray together 1 Peter 1:3-9, and then, with everyone's head bowed, ask if anyone would like to thank God openly for a current circumstance.

week five: God's best for your waiting rooms

Open today's session by acknowledging that no one likes waiting—there will be sighs of agreement. Ask each participant what is hardest for him or her to wait for and how he or she manages (or doesn't manage) the wait. Ask if anyone wants to share how after a long wait for the answer to prayer, the Lord's answer was better than they had anticipated.

On Day One, the group kept track of the time spent waiting in an average day. Share ideas for making waiting times more productive.

Ask a volunteer to read Luke 12:35-48, and discuss answers to the questions regarding this passage. Be sure all understand that the Master is Jesus and ask for sharing of how this parable puts into perspective a current waiting situation.

Discuss the false teachings Christians encounter today and how the group participants can protect themselves from being swayed. Talk about Titus 2:1-8 being the scriptural foundation for Christians mentoring the Christian life to spiritually younger believers and seekers, as Naomi did for Ruth. Discuss the ways Naomi mentored Ruth.

Talk about how this week's lesson has encouraged participants to follow the First Place 4 Health program and wait for their desired weight-loss results, rather than trying fad diets that promise quick weight loss.

Discuss with the group the variety of talents that each participant has. Make the point that everyone has at least one talent. Encourage the group to think beyond typical job descriptions.

Have someone read Psalm 46:10, and invite each person to share one thing he or she is waiting on right now. Follow with a time of group prayer, and after the last amen, ask the group to sit quietly before the Lord for 15 minutes. Ask if anyone felt God impressing something on them that they would like to share.

week six: God's best for your appearance

On Day One, participants explored the values of the world versus God's values. Down the left side of a whiteboard, list things members think the world values most. Then next to each one write what God values most.

The Day Two study looked at how our spiritual heart is at the center of our motives and thoughts. On a whiteboard, list the participants' synonyms for "heart" and "motive." Ask volunteers to finish the phrase "I have my heart set on_____." Have them repeat the phrase substituting a synonym from the board for the word "heart."

Lead a discussion about what a heart could be hungry for instead of food. Emphasize how having Scripture in your heart can nurture your heart in such a way that your physical appearance is transfigured. Ask for ideas about how this happens.

On Day Four, participants studied the world's idea of beauty as opposed to God's idea of beauty. Have participants list the characteristics they found that God values and deems beautiful, and write these responses on the whiteboard.

Talk about how Boaz's actions impressed Ruth. Point out that Boaz was an older man, but Ruth saw that he was a kind man of integrity and generosity. Use this discussion to talk about how we shouldn't judge people by their outward appearance.

week seven: God's best for your attitude

On a whiteboard, compare God's best and Satan's best for your attitude, based on the Scriptures listed in the charts in Day Two.

This is a good time to discuss Day Four's topic on attitude being a choice. Have someone read Romans 7:15-24, and talk about how we all can identify with Paul and his struggles with doing what he didn't want to do—repeatedly sinning. Point out that the reason we keep doing something is because it gives us more satisfaction than honoring God does.

Turn to Ephesians 4:22-24, and ask if anyone feels their attitude about weight and food is the result of something in their past. Remind them that they're new creations in Christ, and help them understand the importance of resolving past issues in order to enjoy the changes they are making as members of this group.

Spend some time discussing the SAT test. Ask volunteers to share how they usually respond in various situations. Go over the biblical ways to respond, and ask the participants to offer practical suggestions for each other. Close your time together with testimonies of how the First Place 4 Health group has helped them make attitude changes. Be sure everyone feels affirmed. Again, offer them the treat and take a bite yourself so that they'll have the assurance that it's safe to eat.

week eight: God's best for your finances

Ask someone to recite from memory Philippians 4:19. Start a discussion of how our management of money relates to our spiritual life, and how needs are not the same as wants. Discuss how God provided for the Israelites' needs but that their desires and cravings caused them to sin.

On Day Two, the discussion mentioned how the media and society feed our hunger to possess more. Ask what tactics are used to inundate us with temptations to buy what we don't need.

Lead a discussion about the difference between Solomon receiving wisdom and God denying wisdom to Adam and Eve. Be sure the participants note that Solomon humbly asked for wisdom to be a better king and that Adam and Eve wanted wisdom for selfish reasons.

Have volunteers read 1 Kings 3:9 and Proverbs 3:21, and as a group, formulate God's definition of wisdom. If it's not mentioned, point out that wisdom comes from the heart, the center of what we treasure most.

Discuss the practicality of the money-management principles. Ask why someone may find following the principles difficult. Then ask for specific suggestions for how the principles *can* be applied. Conclude that regaining financial fitness can be a slow process, but one well worth the effort and time.

Summarize the parable about the rich young man (see Luke 12:16-21), and ask if the group would like to participate in a project to help someone less fortunate by making meals, collecting groceries or creating care packages. Help the group brainstorm ideas of how to use some of their "treasures" to assist God's work at a local shelter.

Ask volunteers to share any other grocery-store traps they know about. Close today's session by reciting in unison the memory verse.

week nine: God's best for your daily life

The spiritual concepts of consecration, or sanctification, may be new to some participants, so be sure everyone knows how these terms apply to the Christian life today. Discuss that ordinary humans are made holy, or sanctified, through Jesus, and we are to set ourselves apart from evil, turning to the Lord and living pure and holy lives ready to serve God. Our holiness should reflect in everything we say and do.

Stress that as we rely on the Holy Spirit and obey God's Word, the Lord helps us become the kind of people He wants us to be. Discuss the struggle Paul talked about in Romans 8:9-17 and why we can't use the excuse "I'm only human" when we sin. Ask the group if they think they're doing a good job in their daily lives of standing out and standing up for God.

Day Four included a discussion about Christians as saints. Ask how knowing that God sees each Christian as a saint affects their daily behavior, treatment of their body, and relationships with others.

The group probably will mention the difficulty in living a holy, set apart life in today's culture. Turn to the Scriptures listed in the chart in Day Four and do a round robin of Scripture reading, offering ways the Scriptures will help the group maintain purity in daily life.

Day Five focused on the amazing things God does in the life of every believer. Be sensitive to anyone in the group struggling with infertility, but discuss God allowing Ruth to have a baby with Boaz, after 10 years of infertility in her first marriage, and God's plans for Ruth to be the great-grandmother of King David. That's a miracle!

Lead a discussion about how this week's lesson has encouraged each First Place 4 Health member to live a holy life, ready and available for God's use. Ask the group for some practical suggestions of what to do when confronted by a social meeting or function that involves activities that go against teachings from the Bible or what to do when they have to interact with people whose values are more worldly than godly.

Close by reminding the group that being holy carries heavy responsibilities in regard to our behavior but that the rewards are worth our following God's leading—"the Lord will do amazing things among you."

week ten: God's best for your service and ministry

This week started out looking at the context of the memory verse and the concept that we'll each have a different body in heaven. Lead a discussion of how this knowledge influences concerns about their earthly body.

The Day Two study encouraged everyone to stand firm and not lose conviction to serve God. Ask what kind of spiritual battles the participants have encountered. Ask if anyone has ever attempted to sway their faith or if any worldly temptation has loosened their footing.

On Day Three, participants looked at service as an *opportunity* rather than an *obligation*. Put the names Naomi, Ruth and Boaz on a whiteboard and list ways participants saw these three seize opportunities to help each other.

Day Four focuses on the potential labor involved in serving God. Stress that God wants us serving with a willing heart, not a duty-bound heart. On a whiteboard write the statements from 2 Corinthians 6:9-10 and 2 Corinthians 4:7-9 and ask group participants if they would like to personalize Paul's statements. For example, "I have nothing, yet I have everything in Christ."

Ask for volunteers to share their descriptions of opportunities for workers of the Lord to serve. Make sure answers include the following: Planters—introducing the good news; Waterers—answering questions or inviting to church and Christian fellowship; Growers—loving, praying and feeding the Word; Harvesters—helping make a decision for Christ.

Day Five should be an encouragement to find God at work and join Him. Do a round robin of reading aloud through the story in John 4:1-42 and answer the questions pertaining to this passage. Introduce the idea that the group might be able to serve together in a community project to help plant and water seeds.

week eleven: God's best for your future

Start by asking if anyone wants to recite the entire 23rd Psalm. If not, read it in unison. Then offer each person a cup of coffee or tea or some other beverage, and ask one participant to keep everyone's cup full throughout the session.

Day One involved a discussion of shepherds and God as the Good Shepherd. On a whiteboard, list answers to the shepherd qualities of King David, God and Jesus. Then read 1 Peter 5:2-3 and discuss the ways Naomi was a shepherd to Ruth. Talk about who each participant should be shepherding and who shepherds them.

On Day Three, participants were reminded that believers are royal priests anointed to do God's work, but sometimes they may feel more like bruised and battered sheep. Ask for volunteers to read aloud the verses in the chart and discuss what "soothing oil" God can provide in times of trouble.

On Day Four, the group considered the literal and metaphorical meanings of "cup." Ask what a cup can hold, according to the Scriptures listed in the chart, and ask how we are to respond to our cup being filled with blessings and joy. Ask if their "cup" has ever been filled with anger or troubles. Have they ever let those things overflow? Emphasize that we have a God who overflows our cup with blessings and joy. Ask for some practical ideas of how to share with others our blessings and joy. Ask a volunteer to read Romans 12:1. Discuss how living out this verse will help fulfill God's best for their future.

Day Five included a description Jesus gave of Himself. Be sure the group understands Jesus' subtle wording change. According to verse 25, believers die to themselves to be reborn here on earth and live a new life in Christ. According to verse 26, believers live eternally.

Lead a discussion of what a refuge is and how God is a refuge for us. Help the group understand that although we have God's goodness (all those blessings and joy), we also need His love (or mercy) because we continue to sin. When we ask for forgiveness for our sins, God, in His love and mercy, cleanses us.

Start a discussion about our eternal dwelling place by stating, "There's no place like home." Ask the group to explain why this adage is true—what does a home usually provide, no matter how long we've been away from it. Then ask how this adage also applies to our heavenly home.

week twelve: time to celebrate!

Even though most of your meeting this week will be a victory celebration, take some time at the beginning of the meeting to talk about how much God loves each person in the group and how each of us is called to love our brothers and sisters in Christ. (See "Planning a Victory Celebration" in the *First Place 4 Health Leader's Guide* for ideas about throwing a successful celebration for your group.)

For the rest of the study time, allow each member to tell his or her *God's best for your life* story. Give members an equal opportunity to share the goals they set for themselves at the beginning of the session and talk about the challenges and good things God has done for them throughout the process. Don't allow the more talkative group members to monopolize all the time. Even the quiet members need an opportunity to share their stories and successes! Even those who have not met their goals have still been part of the journey, so allow them to share and talk about why they did not succeed.

Making a commitment to continue in First Place 4 Health is an important part of victory. Be sure to talk about your group's future plans, and make each person feel welcome to continue to journey with you.

First Place 4 Health menu plans

Each menu plan is based on approximately 1,400 to 1,500 calories per day. All recipe and menu exchanges were determined using the Master-Cook software, a program that accesses a database containing more than 6,000 food items prepared using the United States Department of Agriculture (USDA) publications and information from food manufacturers. As with any nutritional program, MasterCook calculates the nutritional values of the recipes based on ingredients. Nutrition may vary due to how the food is prepared, where the food comes from, soil content, season, ripeness, processing and method of preparation. For these reasons, please use the recipes and menu plans as approximate guides. Consult a physician and/or a registered dietitian before starting a weight-loss program.

For those who need more calories, add the following to the 1,400-calorie plan:

- 1,800 calories: 2 ounce equivalent of meat, 3 ounce equivalent of bread, $^1/_2$ cup vegetable serving, 1 tsp. fat

- 2,000 calories: 2 ounce equivalent of meat, 4 ounce equivalent of bread, $^1/_2$ cup vegetable serving, 3 tsp. fat

- 2,200 calories: 2 ounce equivalent of meat, 5 ounce equivalent of bread, $^1/_2$ cup vegetable serving, $^1/_2$ cup fruit serving, 5 tsp. fat

- 2,400 calories: 2 ounce equivalent of meat, 6 ounce equivalent of bread, 1 cup vegetable serving, $^1/_2$ cup fruit serving, 6 tsp. fat

First Week Grocery List

Produce

- [ ] apple
- [ ] asparagus spears
- [ ] baby carrots
- [ ] basil
- [ ] bell pepper
- [ ] blackberries
- [ ] broccoli
- [ ] carrots
- [ ] celery
- [ ] cilantro
- [ ] corn
- [ ] eggplant
- [ ] garlic cloves
- [ ] grapes
- [ ] grapefruit
- [ ] lemon juice
- [ ] lemons
- [ ] lettuce
- [ ] lime juice
- [ ] melon
- [ ] mushrooms
- [ ] onion
- [ ] oregano
- [ ] oranges
- [ ] peaches
- [ ] pears
- [ ] pineapple
- [ ] raisins
- [ ] raspberries
- [ ] red onion
- [ ] red potatoes
- [ ] salad
- [ ] strawberries
- [ ] sugar snap peas
- [ ] tomatoes
- [ ] watermelon
- [ ] zucchini

Condiments/Spreads

- [ ] fig preserves
- [ ] mayonnaise, light
- [ ] Ranch dressing, light
- [ ] salad dressing, light
- [ ] salsa, chunky
- [ ] soy sauce
- [ ] sweet pickle relish

Breads, Cereals and Pasta

- [ ] bagels
- [ ] bread, cinnamon-raisin
- [ ] bread, whole-wheat
- [ ] breadsticks
- [ ] brown rice
- [ ] cornflakes
- [ ] English muffin
- [ ] lasagna noodles, no-bake
- [ ] Melba toast
- [ ] oatmeal
- [ ] rice pilaf
- [ ] saltine crackers
- [ ] spaghetti

Canned Foods

- [ ] all-vegetable soup
- [ ] black beans
- [ ] diced tomatoes with chilies
- [ ] Italian-style tomatoes with peppers
- [ ] spaghetti sauce

- [ ] tomato sauce
- [ ] tomato soup, low-sodium
- [ ] tuna, water-packed
- [ ] whole tomatoes, no-salt-added

Dairy Products
- [ ] cheese, 2% cheddar
- [ ] cheese, mozzarella
- [ ] cheese, Parmesan
- [ ] cheese, Parmigiano-Reggiano
- [ ] cheese, Provolone, reduced-fat
- [ ] cheese, ricotta
- [ ] cheese, Swiss
- [ ] cottage cheese, 2%
- [ ] goat cheese
- [ ] margarine
- [ ] milk, skim
- [ ] yogurt, vanilla low-fat

Juices
- [ ] orange juice
- [ ] pineapple juice

Frozen Foods
- [ ] pancakes
- [ ] peas
- [ ] spinach
- [ ] Stouffer's Beef Stroganoff Casserole®
- [ ] waffles, whole-grain

Meat and Poultry
- [ ] chicken, boneless and skinless
- [ ] eggs
- [ ] fish fillets
- [ ] ham, lean
- [ ] Italian turkey sausage links
- [ ] turkey

First Week Meals and Recipes

DAY 1

....

Breakfast

Whole-grain Waffles with Berries and Yogurt Dressing

2 cups vanilla low-fat yogurt	$1/3$ cup sugar
2 tbsp. honey	2 tbsp. fresh lemon juice
2 cups fresh raspberries	4 frozen whole-grain waffles,
1 cup quartered small strawberries	toasted
1 cup fresh blackberries	4 tsp. toasted wheat germ

Drain yogurt in a fine sieve or colander lined with cheesecloth for 10 minutes and then spoon into a bowl. Add honey and stir to combine. Combine berries, sugar and juice, and then let stand for 5 minutes. Place 1 waffle on each of 4 plates and top each serving with 1 cup fruit mixture, about $1/3$ cup yogurt mixture, and 1 teaspoon wheat germ. Serve immediately. Serves 4.

Nutritional Information: 354 calories; 5g fat (12.3% calories from fat); 9g protein; 71g carbohydrate; 8g dietary fiber; 17mg cholesterol; 338mg sodium.

....

Lunch

2 cups all-vegetable soup	1 orange
6 saltine crackers	

Nutritional Information: 284 calories; 6g fat (18.8% calories from fat); 7g protein; 52g carbohydrate; 5g dietary fiber; 0mg cholesterol; 1,878mg sodium.

....

Dinner

Southwestern-Style Baked Fish with Black Bean Salsa

Salsa

1 16-oz. can black beans, drained	1 cup chunky salsa
1 tbsp. red onion, diced	1 tbsp. fresh cilantro, chopped
1 tsp. chili powder	

Fish

4 4-oz. fish filets	$^1/_2$ tsp. ground cumin
2 tsp. lime juice	nonstick cooking spray
salt and black pepper	

Combine salsa ingredients in small bowl and set aside. Coat a 9″ x 9″ baking pan with nonstick cooking spray. Season filets, place in a pan and bake at 400° F for 12 to 15 minutes (10 minutes per inch of thickness). Garnish with salsa. Serve with $^1/_3$ cup rice, one 6-inch ear of corn and 1 cup steamed broccoli with 1 teaspoon melted margarine. Serves 4.

Nutritional Information: 551 calories; 6g fat (8.9% calories from fat); 37g protein; 90g carbohydrate; 13g dietary fiber; 49mg cholesterol; 780mg sodium.

DAY 2

Breakfast

1 whole-grain English muffin	$^1/_2$ grapefruit
1 egg, poached	

Nutritional Information: 246 calories; 6g fat (22.7% calories from fat); 13g protein; 37g carbohydrate; 5g dietary fiber; 212mg cholesterol; 560mg sodium.

Lunch

Tuna Melt

$^1/_2$ cup water-packed tuna	2 slices whole-wheat bread
1 tbsp. light mayonnaise	1 slice reduced-fat Provolone
$^1/_2$ tsp. sweet pickle relish	or Swiss cheese

Mix tuna, mayonnaise and relish together and spread on one slice of toasted bread. Top with cheese and broil until the cheese is melted. Top with the other slice of toasted bread and serve with 1 cup diced watermelon. Serves 1.

Nutritional Information: 517 calories; 12g fat (21.3% calories from fat); 58g protein; 44g carbohydrate; 5g dietary fiber; 68mg cholesterol; 948mg sodium.

Dinner

Spicy Eggplant Casserole

2 small eggplants, peeled and cut	$1^1/_2$ tbsp. onion, chopped
into 1-inch cubes	$1^1/_2$ tbsp. celery, chopped

1¹/₂ tbsp. bell pepper, chopped
1 10-oz. can diced tomatoes
  with chilies
cayenne pepper

salt
¹/₂ cup soft bread cubes
2 oz. 2% cheddar cheese, shredded
nonstick cooking spray

Salt eggplant and let sit for 20 minutes to draw out the bitterness. Rinse and drain. Combine eggplant, onion, celery, bell pepper, tomatoes with chilies, salt, cayenne pepper and bread cubes in bowl and pour into a 9″ x 9″ baking dish coated with nonstick cooking spray. Top with cheese and bake at 400° F for 20 to 25 minutes. Serve with a green salad with light dressing and a breadstick. Serves 4.

Nutritional Information: 329 calories; 11g fat (29.5% calories from fat); 31g protein; 29g carbohydrate; 9g dietary fiber; 53mg cholesterol; 427mg sodium.

DAY 3

Breakfast

Grilled Goat Cheese Sandwich with Fig Preserves

2 tsp. honey
¹/₄ tsp. grated lemon rind
1 (4-oz.) package goat cheese
2 tbsp. fig preserves

8 (1-oz.) slices cinnamon-
  raisin bread
1 tsp. powdered sugar
nonstick cooking spray

Combine honey, lemon rind and goat cheese, stirring until well blended. Spread 1 tablespoon of the goat cheese mixture on each of the 4 bread slices, and then top each slice with 1¹/₂ teaspoons preserves. Top with the remaining bread slices. Lightly coat the outside of the bread with nonstick cooking spray. Heat a large nonstick skillet over medium heat and add 2 sandwiches to the pan. Press gently to flatten. Cook for 3 minutes on each side or until the bread is lightly toasted. Repeat with remaining sandwiches and sprinkle with sugar. Serves 4.

Nutritional Information: 307 calories; 13g fat (33.6% calories from fat); 13g protein; 46g carbohydrate; 1g dietary fiber; 30mg cholesterol; 298mg sodium.

Lunch

Bagel Sandwich

2 oz. turkey, sliced

1 (2-oz.) bagel, spread with 1 tsp. light
  mayonnaise lettuce and tomato

Serve with 1 cup carrots with 2 tbsp. light Ranch dressing.

Nutritional Information: 329 calories; 7g fat (18.2% calories from fat); 17g protein; 50g carbohydrate; 6g dietary fiber; 32mg cholesterol; 440mg sodium.

....

Dinner

Vegetable Lasagna

6 no-bake lasagna noodles	2 eggs, slightly beaten
2 tbsp. canola oil	2 cups ricotta cheese
1 cup onion, chopped	4 tbsp. Parmesan cheese
1¹/₂ cups carrots, sliced thin	1 cup mushrooms, sliced
2 tsp. garlic, minced	1 tsp. leaf basil
1 (15-oz.) jar spaghetti sauce	¹/₂ tsp. leaf oregano
1 cup zucchini, quartered and sliced	1 (10-oz.) package frozen chopped
1 cup part-skim mozzarella cheese,	spinach, thawed and drained
shredded	nonstick cooking spray

Heat oil in a saucepan and add onion, carrots and garlic. Sauté for 5 to 6 minutes or until the vegetables are tender. Add sauce and spices and bring to a simmer. Blend eggs with ricotta cheese, Parmesan cheese and vegetables. Spread a thin layer of sauce on the bottom of a 9″ x 11″ baking pan coated with nonstick cooking spray. Cover with a layer of noodles and then spoon half the cheese-vegetable mixture over noodles. Cover with half of the remaining sauce. Repeat. Cover with foil and bake at 350° F for 20 minutes. Remove foil and top with mozzarella cheese, and then bake uncovered for 15 minutes. Let sit for 10 minutes before slicing. Serve each slice with a 3-inch French bread with 1 teaspoon margarine, a tossed salad with reduced fat dressing, and a cup of fruit salad. Serves 6.

Nutritional Information: 561 calories; 15g fat (22.7% calories from fat); 19g protein; 92g carbohydrate; 9g dietary fiber; 58mg cholesterol; 530mg sodium.

DAY 4

....

Breakfast

³/₄ cup corn flakes	1 cup skim milk
¹/₂ small bagel, toasted	1 cup mixed melon cubes
1 tsp. light margarine	

Nutritional Information: 293 calories; 4g fat (11.7% calories from fat); 12g protein; 56g carbohydrate; 5g dietary fiber; 4mg cholesterol; 322mg sodium.

Lunch

Chick-fil-A Chargrilled Chicken
Sandwich®

Side of carrot and raisin salad
$1/_2$ cup grapes

Nutritional Information: 490 calories; 22g fat (26.2% calories from fat); 31g protein; 105g carbohydrate; 8g dietary fiber; 65mg cholesterol; 1,351mg sodium.

Dinner

Chicken Cacciatore

1 (2$1/_2$-lb.) skinless chicken,
  quartered with skin removed
1 (16-oz.) can Italian-style tomatoes
  with peppers

1 onion, sliced
1 tsp. Italian herb seasoning
1 (8-oz.) can tomato sauce
2 cups frozen peas

Spray a large saucepan with nonstick cooking spray and add chicken, tomatoes with peppers, onion, Italian herb seasoning and tomato sauce. Cover and simmer for 25 to 35 minutes, stirring occasionally. Add the peas and cook for an additional 10 minutes. Serve each with $1/_2$ cup boiled red potatoes and $1/_2$ cup steamed baby carrots. Serves 4.

Nutritional Information: 532 calories; 5g fat (9.1% calories from fat); 74g protein; 44g carbohydrate; 10g dietary fiber; 165mg cholesterol; 921mg sodium.

DAY 5

Breakfast

1 cup oatmeal with $1/_2$ tsp.
  cinnamon and $1/_4$ cup raisins

1 cup skim milk

Nutritional Information: 335 calories; 3g fat (7.7% calories from fat); 15g protein; 65g carbohydrate; 6g dietary fiber; 4mg cholesterol; 508mg sodium.

Lunch

1 cup low-sodium tomato soup
1 cup celery sticks
6 slices Melba toast

$1/_2$ cup 2% cottage cheese
$1/_3$ cup peach slices

Nutritional Information: 257 calories; 3g fat (10.3% calories from fat); 21g protein; 39g carbohydrate; 7g dietary fiber; 9mg cholesterol; 1,598mg sodium.

Dinner

Stouffer's Beef Stroganoff Casserole®

Serve with a spinach salad with mushrooms and light salad dressing and a peach.

Nutritional Information: 446 calories; 18g fat (34.9% calories from fat); 25g protein; 49g carbohydrate; 6g dietary fiber; 70mg cholesterol; 1,048mg sodium.

DAY 6

Breakfast

3 4-inch low-fat pancakes   1 cup skim milk
1 tbsp. light syrup
1 cup strawberries, sliced

Nutritional Information: 356 calories; 4g fat (9.8% calories from fat); 15g protein; 65g carbohydrate; 5g dietary fiber; 18mg cholesterol; 844mg sodium.

Lunch

Ham, Asparagus and Rice Rolls

2 oz. lean ham, sliced thin $^1/_2$ cup cooked brown rice
4 large asparagus spears, cooked

Wrap ham around asparagus spears and rice. Serve with 1 pear.

Nutritional Information: 325 calories; 8g fat (20.3% calories from fat); 14g protein; 53g carbohydrate; 7g dietary fiber; 32mg cholesterol; 749mg sodium.

Dinner

Easy Spaghetti with Sausage

8 oz. hot Italian turkey sausage links   5 garlic cloves, minced
8 oz. uncooked spaghetti   1 tsp. sugar
1 (28-oz.) can no-salt-added whole $^1/_2$ tsp. salt
  tomatoes, undrained $^1/_4$ cup torn fresh basil
2 tbsp. olive oil $^1/_2$ cup (2 oz.) shaved Parmigiano-
$^1/_2$ tsp. crushed red pepper   Reggiano cheese

Preheat broiler. Arrange sausage on a small baking sheet. Broil sausage for 5 minutes on each side or until done. Remove the pan from oven (do not turn the broiler off) and cut the sausage into $1/4$-inch-thick slices. Arrange the slices in a single layer on baking sheet. Broil the sausage slices for 2 minutes or until browned. Cook pasta according to package directions, omitting salt and fat, and drain. Place the tomatoes in a food processor and process until almost smooth. Heat the olive oil in a large skillet over medium-high heat. Add crushed red pepper and minced garlic and sauté for 1 minute. Stir in tomatoes, sugar and salt and cook 4 minutes or until slightly thick. Add the sausage and cooked pasta to the pan and toss well. Top with fresh basil and Parmigiano-Reggiano. Serve with mixed green salad and light dressing. Serves 4.

Nutritional Information: 442 calories; 19g fat (38.1% calories from fat); 21g protein; 47g carbohydrate; 2g dietary fiber; 54mg cholesterol; 998mg sodium.

DAY 7

Breakfast

Orange Cranberry Muffins

1 $1/2$ cups all-purpose flour (about 6 $3/4$ oz.)	$1/8$ tsp. ground nutmeg
$1/2$ cup raw wheat germ	$3/4$ cup packed brown sugar
$1/2$ cup sweetened dried cranberries	$1/4$ cup canola oil
1 tsp. baking powder	1 tsp. grated orange rind
$1/2$ tsp. baking soda	$1/2$ cup fresh orange juice
$1/2$ tsp. ground cinnamon	2 large eggs
$1/4$ tsp. salt	1 tbsp. sugar
	nonstick cooking spray

Preheat oven to 375° F. Lightly spoon flour into dry measuring cups and level with a knife. Combine flour, wheat germ, cranberries, baking powder, baking soda, cinnamon, salt and nutmeg in a large bowl and stir with a whisk. Make a well in the center of the mixture. Combine brown sugar, oil, orange rind, orange juice and eggs in a bowl and stir with a whisk. Add the egg mixture to the flour mixture and stir just until combined. Spoon batter into 12 muffin cups coated with cooking spray and then sprinkle with sugar. Bake at 375° F for 17 minutes or until muffins spring back when touched in the center. (*Note*: These muffins freeze great.) Serves 12.

Nutritional Information: 188 calories; 6g fat (28.4% calories from fat); 4g protein; 30g carbohydrate; 1g dietary fiber; 35mg cholesterol; 156mg sodium.

Lunch

Arby's Junior Roast Beef Sandwich®   1 tbsp. reduced-fat dressing
dark green salad with veggies   1 small apple

Nutritional Information: 436 calories; 16g fat (31.6% calories from fat); 19g protein; 60g carbohydrate; 8g dietary fiber; 31mg cholesterol; 911mg sodium.

Dinner

Grilled Hawaiian Chicken

4 4-oz. boneless chicken breasts with $^1/_2$ cup cooking sherry
  skin   1 tsp. brown sugar
$^1/_2$ cup pineapple juice   8 fresh pineapple slices
$^1/_4$ cup soy sauce

Place chicken in a glass bowl. Combine pineapple juice, soy sauce, cooking sherry, brown sugar and pineapple slices in a bowl. Pour the mixture over the chicken breasts and marinate overnight (or up to 48 hours). Remove the breasts and grill over medium heat until done. Remove the skin before serving. Grill fresh pineapple slices for garnish. Serve each with $^2/_3$ cup rice pilaf and 1 cup sautéed sugar snap peas. Serves 4.

Nutritional Information: 452 calories; 4g fat (9.1% calories from fat); 34g protein; 62g carbohydrate; 5g dietary fiber; 72mg cholesterol; 1,660mg sodium.

Second Week Grocery List

Produce
- ❑ apples
- ❑ apricots
- ❑ baby carrots
- ❑ baby spinach
- ❑ broccoli
- ❑ carrots
- ❑ cauliflower
- ❑ cherry tomatoes
- ❑ cucumbers
- ❑ eggplant
- ❑ fruit salad
- ❑ garlic
- ❑ green bell peppers
- ❑ green onions
- ❑ lemons
- ❑ lemon juice
- ❑ mushrooms
- ❑ onions
- ❑ orange
- ❑ pears
- ❑ peppers
- ❑ pineapple
- ❑ plum tomatoes
- ❑ potatoes
- ❑ red onion
- ❑ spring mix salad greens
- ❑ shallots
- ❑ strawberries
- ❑ summer squash
- ❑ tomatoes
- ❑ zucchini

Baking/Cooking Products
- ❑ all-purpose flour
- ❑ balsamic vinegar
- ❑ basil
- ❑ black beans
- ❑ black pepper
- ❑ brown mustard
- ❑ brown sugar
- ❑ canola oil
- ❑ dill
- ❑ garlic, granulated
- ❑ herbed stuffing mix
- ❑ lemon pepper seasoning
- ❑ nonstick cooking spray (butter flavored)
- ❑ olive oil
- ❑ oregano
- ❑ paprika
- ❑ salt
- ❑ thyme
- ❑ white wine vinegar

Condiments/Spreads
- ❑ all-fruit spread, strawberry
- ❑ Italian dressing, light
- ❑ peanut butter
- ❑ Ranch dressing, light
- ❑ salad dressing, fat-free
- ❑ salsa
- ❑ Worcestershire sauce

Breads and Cereals
- ❑ bagels, sesame
- ❑ bread, whole-wheat
- ❑ breadsticks
- ❑ dinner rolls
- ❑ English muffin

- ❏ French bread
- ❏ graham crackers
- ❏ granola bar, low-fat
- ❏ grits
- ❏ Italian bread
- ❏ pita chips
- ❏ rice
- ❏ saltine crackers
- ❏ tortillas, corn
- ❏ tortillas, fat-free flour
- ❏ tortilla chips

Canned Foods
- ❏ Campbell's Chunky Manhattan-Style Clam Chowder®
- ❏ chicken broth
- ❏ cinnamon applesauce

Dairy Products
- ❏ blue cheese
- ❏ cheese, reduced-fat cheddar
- ❏ cheese, reduced-fat sharp cheddar
- ❏ cheese, reduced-sodium Muenster
- ❏ cheese, Parmesan
- ❏ cheese, Parmigiano-Reggiano
- ❏ cream cheese, fat-free

- ❏ milk, skim
- ❏ sour cream, fat-free
- ❏ yogurt, nonfat fruit flavored

Juices
- ❏ orange juice

Frozen Foods
- ❏ Healthy Choice Ginger Chicken®
- ❏ peas
- ❏ waffles, low-fat

Meat and Poultry
- ❏ Canadian bacon
- ❏ chicken breasts, boneless, skinless
- ❏ deli ham
- ❏ deli roast beef, low-sodium
- ❏ eggs
- ❏ egg substitute
- ❏ halibut filets
- ❏ ham
- ❏ shrimp, precooked
- ❏ sirloin, lean
- ❏ turkey
- ❏ turkey mignons

Second Week Meals and Recipes

DAY 1

Breakfast

2 oz. sesame bagel
1 tbsp. fat-free cream cheese

$^1/_2$ cup orange juice
6 oz. nonfat fruit-flavored yogurt

Nutritional Information: 311 calories; 2g fat (4.7% calories from fat); 16g protein; 58g carbohydrate; 2g dietary fiber; 3mg cholesterol; 479mg sodium.

Lunch

Grilled Ham and Muenster

8 slices Italian bread ($^1/_2$ inch thick)
8 oz. thin sliced lower-sodium deli ham
2 cups fresh baby spinach

4 (1-oz.) slices reduced-sodium
    Muenster cheese
nonstick cooking spray

Layer the 4 bread slices with 2 ounces ham, 1 slice Muenster cheese and $^1/_2$ cup baby spinach. Top with remaining bread slices. Heat a large nonstick skillet over medium-high heat. Coat sandwiches with nonstick cooking spray and add to pan. Cook for 2 minutes on each side or until the sandwiches are browned and the cheese melts. Serve immediately. Serves 4.

Nutritional Information: 314 calories; 10g fat (31.1% calories from fat); 22g protein; 30g carbohydrate; 2g dietary fiber; 57mg cholesterol; 1,342mg sodium.

Dinner

Campbell's Chunky Manhattan-Style
    Clam Chowder®
dark green salad

cucumbers, carrots and tomatoes
fat-free dressing
French bread slice

Nutritional Information: 357 calories; 8g fat (20% calories from fat); 15g protein; 61g carbohydrate; 10g dietary fiber; 10mg cholesterol; 1,867mg sodium.

DAY 2

Breakfast
Spanish Omelet

$^1/_2$ cup egg substitute
$^1/_4$ cup tomatoes, diced

1 tsp. onions, diced
1 tsp. peppers, diced

Spray small frying pan with nonstick cooking spray. Combine egg substitute, tomatoes, onions and peppers and cook over medium heat until done. Serve with 1 slice whole-wheat toast and $^1/_2$ cup fresh pineapple.

Nutritional Information: 310 calories; 15g fat (42.4% calories from fat); 17g protein; 29g carbohydrate; 3g dietary fiber; 2mg cholesterol; 392mg sodium.

Lunch
Healthy Choice Ginger Chicken® $^1/_2$ cup mixed fruit salad

Nutritional Information: 433 calories; 5g fat (9.7% calories from fat); 16g protein; 83g carbohydrate; 5g dietary fiber; 25mg cholesterol; 314mg sodium.

Dinner
Chicken Ratatouille
4 4-oz. boneless, skinless chicken breasts, cubed	1 green bell peppers, sliced
1 small eggplant, cubed	1 large tomato, cubed
2 small zucchini, sliced	$^1/_2$ tsp. leaf thyme
1 onion, sliced	1 tsp. leaf basil
$^1/_2$ lb. mushrooms, sliced	1 tbsp. olive oil
$^1/_2$ tsp. granulated garlic	1 tsp. black pepper

In a large saucepan, sauté chicken in olive oil (about 2 minutes per side). Add eggplant, zucchini, onion, mushrooms and bell pepper. Simmer for 10 minutes and then add tomato, thyme, basil, olive oil and black pepper. Simmer for 3 to 5 minutes. Serve each with $^2/_3$ cup cooked rice and a Caesar salad with light dressing. Serves 4.

Nutritional Information: 425 calories; 6g fat (13.3% calories from fat); 36g protein; 58g carbohydrate; 9g dietary fiber; 66mg cholesterol; 128mg sodium.

DAY 3

Breakfast
$^1/_2$ cup cooked grits	1 slice whole-wheat bread
1 oz. reduced-fat cheddar cheese, shredded	1 tsp. all-fruit spread
	$^1/_2$ cup orange juice

Nutritional Information: 293 calories; 4g fat (11.7% calories from fat); 12g protein; 56g carbohydrate; 5g dietary fiber; 4mg cholesterol; 322mg sodium.

Lunch

2 tbsp. peanut butter
4 graham cracker squares
1 apple, sliced

1 cup broccoli florets with
1 tbsp. light Ranch dressing

Nutritional Information: 354 calories; 19g fat (44.2% calories from fat); 11g protein; 42g carbohydrate; 8g dietary fiber; trace cholesterol; 264mg sodium.

Dinner

Grilled or Broiled Halibut

4 4-oz. halibut filets
2 tbsp. light Italian dressing
2 tsp. Worcestershire sauce

$1/_2$ tsp. paprika
$1/_4$ tsp. black pepper

Combine all ingredients in a 9″ x 9″ baking dish. Let marinate for 30 minutes in the refrigerator. Grill or broil fish about 10 minutes per inch of thickness (about 5 minutes per side). Serve each with $1/_2$ cup mashed potatoes, 1 cup assorted grilled vegetables and a dinner roll. Serves 4.

Nutritional Information: 304 calories; 8g fat (23.3% calories from fat); 28g protein; 29g carbohydrate; 3g dietary fiber; 39mg cholesterol; 538mg sodium.

DAY 4

Breakfast

1 *Orange Cranberry Muffin* (from last
   week)

1 cup skim milk
$1/_2$ cup cinnamon applesauce

Nutritional Information: 370 calories; 7g fat (15.8% calories from fat); 12g protein; 68g carbohydrate; 3g dietary fiber; 40mg cholesterol; 286mg sodium.

Lunch

Chef's Salad

1 oz. turkey, sliced into thin strips
1 oz. lean ham, sliced into thin strips
2 cups mixed salad greens

tomatoes, carrots and cucumbers
2 tbsp. light dressing

Serve with 2 small breadsticks and 1 pear.

Nutritional Information: 283 calories; 7g fat (21.9% calories from fat); 14g protein; 44g carbohydrate; 8g dietary fiber; 32mg cholesterol; 521mg sodium.

Dinner

Beef Kabobs

1 lb. lean sirloin, cut into 1-inch cubes	2 tsp. olive oil
1 small red onion, quartered	2 tsp. Worcestershire sauce
1 green bell pepper	$1/2$ tsp. oregano
8 mushroom caps	$1/4$ tsp. black pepper
1 zucchini, cut into 12 rounds	12 cherry tomatoes
	nonstick cooking spray

On a wooden or metal skewer, alternate meat and vegetables, except for the cherry tomatoes. Place in a glass dish. In a small bowl combine oil, Worcestershire sauce, oregano and pepper. Pour over kebabs and let marinate covered in refrigerator overnight. Grill to desired doneness and garnish with cherry tomatoes. Serve each with $1/2$ cup grilled red potatoes, a slice of toasted French bread and $1/2$ cup boiled baby carrots sprayed with nonstick (butter-flavored) cooking spray.

Nutritional Information: 480 calories; 20g fat (36.7% calories from fat); 29g protein; 48g carbohydrate; 7g dietary fiber; 71mg cholesterol; 291mg sodium.

DAY 5

Breakfast

2 low-fat waffles	1 cup strawberries, sliced
2 tsp. strawberry all-fruit spread	1 cup skim milk

Nutritional Information: 333 calories; 6g fat (17.1% calories from fat); 13g protein; 56g carbohydrate; 5g dietary fiber; 27mg cholesterol; 654mg sodium.

Lunch

Roast Beef Quesadillas

$1/3$ cup thinly sliced red onion	2 tbsp. crumbled blue cheese
4 (8-inch) fat-free flour tortillas	4 tsp. *Balsamic Glaze*
$1/2$ pound thinly sliced low-sodium deli roast beef	nonstick cooking spray

Heat a large nonstick skillet over medium heat. Coat pan with nonstick cooking spray and add onion. Sauté for 3 to 4 minutes or until tender and lightly browned. Remove from heat. Top half of each tortilla evenly with beef, onion and cheese. Fold the tortillas in half. Return the pan to the heat. Coat the pan and both sides of quesadillas evenly with nonstick cooking spray. Place 2 of the quesadillas in a pan and cook for 2 to 3 minutes on each side or until browned. Repeat procedure with remaining quesadillas. Cut each quesadilla into 4 wedges and drizzle with 1 teaspoon glaze. Serve with 1 ounce baked tortilla chips and salsa. Serves 4.

Balsamic Glaze
1 cup balsamic vinegar   1 tbsp. brown sugar

Mix balsamic vinegar and brown sugar in a skillet. Simmer over low heat until thick (about 20 minutes).

Nutritional Information: 237 calories; 4g fat (14.9% calories from fat); 20g protein; 30g carbohydrate; 6g dietary fiber; 26mg cholesterol; 1,113mg sodium.

Dinner

Chicken Milanese
$3/4$ tsp. fresh lemon juice   2 tbsp. grated Parmigiano-Reggiano
$3/4$ tsp. white wine vinegar   2 tbsp. all-purpose flour
$1/2$ tsp. minced shallots   1 egg white, lightly beaten
$1/4$ tsp. salt $1/4$ tsp. black pepper, divided
dash of sugar   5 tsp. olive oil, divided
2 (6-oz.) skinless, boneless chicken   2 cups packed spring mix salad
   breasts   greens
$1/3$ cup dry breadcrumbs   2 lemon wedges

Combine juice, vinegar, shallots, $1/8$ teaspoon salt and sugar and let stand 15 minutes. Place chicken between 2 sheets of heavy-duty plastic wrap and then pound to $1/2$-inch thickness using a meat mallet or small heavy skillet. Combine the breadcrumbs and cheese in a shallow dish. Place flour in a shallow dish. Place egg white in a shallow dish. Sprinkle the chicken with $1/8$ teaspoon salt and $1/8$ teaspoon pepper. Dredge the chicken in flour, then dip in the egg white, and then dredge in the breadcrumb mixture. Place the chicken on a wire rack and let stand for 5 minutes. Heat 1 tablespoon oil in a large nonstick skillet over medium-high heat. Add chicken and cook for 3 minutes. Turn the chicken over and cook for 2 minutes or until browned and done. Add 2 teaspoons oil and $1/8$ teaspoon pepper to shallot mixture, and then stir with a whisk. Add greens and toss gently. Place 1 chicken breast half and 1 cup salad on each of 2 plates. Serve with lemon wedges. Serves 2.

Nutritional Information: 338 calories; 15g fat (40.2% calories from fat); 28g protein; 23g carbohydrate; 2g dietary fiber; 53mg cholesterol; 581mg sodium.

DAY 6

Breakfast
English Muffin Sandwich
1 English muffin   1 slice tomato
1 oz. Canadian bacon, sautéed

Serve with 1 small orange.

Nutritional Information: 266 calories; 4g fat (12.4% calories from fat); 14g protein; 48g carbohydrate; 9g dietary fiber; 14mg cholesterol; 831mg sodium.

Lunch
1 small low-fat granola bar   2 oz. reduced-fat cheddar cheese
6 saltine crackers   4 canned apricot halves

Nutritional Information: 335 calories; 9g fat (24.1% calories from fat); 18g protein; 46g carbohydrate; 4g dietary fiber; 12mg cholesterol; 667mg sodium.

Dinner
Turkey Steak
4 (3-oz.) turkey mignons $1/2$ cup light Ranch dressing
1 tsp. canola oil   1 tbsp. brown mustard
2 tsp. lemon-pepper seasoning $1/4$ tsp. dill

Heat oil in a large pan. Add mignons and sauté over medium heat for 8 to 10 minutes, turning occasionally. Add lemon-pepper seasoning and sauté for 1 minute more on each side. Combine Ranch dressing, brown mustard and dill to use as a sauce. Serve with 1 cup steamed cauliflower topped with a small amount of the sauce and $1/2$ cup prepared herbed stuffing mix. Serves 4.

Nutritional Information: 438 calories; 19g fat (38.2% calories from fat); 26g protein; 42g carbohydrate; 6g dietary fiber; 56mg cholesterol; 824mg sodium.

DAY 7

....

Breakfast

Quick Breakfast Tostada

1/4 cup 1% low-fat milk
1/4 tsp. salt
1/8 tsp. freshly ground black pepper
4 large egg whites
2 large eggs
4 (6-inch) corn tortillas
1/4 cup chopped green onions

1/2 cup (2 oz.) shredded reduced-fat
   sharp cheddar cheese
1 cup canned black beans, rinsed
   and drained
1/2 cup bottled salsa
1/4 cup fat-free sour cream

Combine milk, salt, black pepper, egg whites and eggs in a large microwave-safe dish, stirring with a whisk. Microwave on high for 3 minutes, and then stir. Microwave the mixture for an additional 1 minute or until done. Arrange 1 tortilla on each of 4 microwave-safe plates and divide egg mixture evenly among the corn tortillas. Layer each serving with 2 tablespoons cheese, 1/4 cup beans and 1 tablespoon green onions. Microwave each tostada on high for 30 seconds. Top each tostada with 2 tablespoons salsa and 1 tablespoon sour cream. Serve immediately. Serves 4.

Nutritional Information: 216 calories; 5g fat (20.3% calories from fat); 17g protein; 26g carbohydrate; 5g dietary fiber; 111mg cholesterol; 710mg sodium.

....

Lunch

McDonald's Hamburger Happy
   Meal®

small diet drink
green salad with light dressing

Nutritional Information: 500 calories; 20g fat (29.4% calories from fat); 17g protein; 92g carbohydrate; 7g dietary fiber; 25mg cholesterol; 719mg sodium.

....

Dinner

Shrimp and Vegetable Risotto

3/4 lb. precooked shrimp
2 tbsp. olive oil, divided
6 plum tomatoes, quartered and
   seeded
1 medium zucchini, cubed

1 medium summer squash, cubed
1 cup mushrooms, sliced
1 cup onions, chopped
1 clove garlic, minced
1 tsp. oregano

3 cups chicken broth
$^3/_4$ cup rice
$^1/_4$ cup Parmesan cheese, grated

salt and pepper
$^1/_2$ cup frozen peas, thawed

Heat oil in a large pan. Add vegetables and sauté over medium heat until crisp tender. Add shrimp and keep warm. In a separate saucepan, add oregano, broth and rice and bring to a boil. Simmer until thickened, stirring occasionally. Stir in Parmesan cheese and season with salt and pepper. In a large bowl, combine shrimp mixture with rice mixture. Toss and garnish with peas. Serve with toasted pita chips. Serves 4.

Nutritional Information: 398 calories; 11g fat (25.1% calories from fat); 30g protein; 44g carbohydrate; 5g dietary fiber; 170mg cholesterol; 900mg sodium.

HEALTHY SNACK CHOICES
(**Note:** Add the ingredients for each of these items to the grocery lists.)

- $3^1/_2$ cups low-fat popcorn topped with 2 tbsp. shredded Parmesan cheese (100 calories)
- 1 cheese stick plus $^1/_2$ cup cherry or grape tomatoes (94 calories)
- 1 bag Baked Cheetos® (100 calories)
- 15 rice crackers (110 calories)
- 1 cup unshelled edamame (120 calories)
- 50 Vegetable Chips (130 calories)
- 1 (1-oz.) package of almonds (130 calories)
- 1 (12-oz.) bottle of V-8® (70 calories plus 3 grams of fiber and 3 servings of vegetables)

ADDITIONAL RECIPES
Cucumber Boats
1 medium-size cucumber
1 tsp. finely chopped parsley
$^1/_4$ tsp. finely chopped basil

$^1/_2$ tsp. finely chopped chives
$^3/_4$ cup low-fat, low-sodium cottage
   cheese

Cut cucumber in half lengthwise. Hollow the center of each cucumber half by scooping out seeds with a spoon. Stir finely chopped herbs into cottage cheese, and then arrange in hollowed cucumbers. Serves 2.

Nutritional Information: 82 calories; 1g fat (11.7% calories from fat); 12g protein; 7g carbohydrate; 1g dietary fiber; 4mg cholesterol; 348mg sodium.

Fresh Tomato Soup

2 cups fat-free, less-sodium chicken broth

1 cup chopped onion

$^3/_4$ cup chopped celery

1 tbsp. thinly sliced fresh basil

1 tbsp. tomato paste

2 pounds plum tomatoes, cut into wedges

$^1/_2$ tsp. salt

$^1/_4$ tsp. freshly ground black pepper

6 tbsp. plain low-fat yogurt

3 tbsp. thinly sliced fresh basil

Combine chicken broth, onion, celery, basil, tomato paste and tomatoes in a large saucepan and bring to a boil. Reduce heat and simmer for 30 minutes. Place half of tomato mixture into a blender. Remove the center piece of the blender lid (to allow steam to escape) and secure the blender lid on blender. Place a clean towel over the opening in the blender lid (to avoid splatters) and blend until smooth. Pour into a large bowl. Repeat procedure with remaining tomato mixture. Stir in salt and pepper. Ladle $^3/_4$ cup soup into each of 6 bowls and top each serving with 1 tablespoon yogurt and 1 $^1/_2$ teaspoons basil. Serves 6.

Nutritional Information: 60 calories; 1g fat (10.4% calories from fat); 4g protein; 11g carbohydrate; 2g dietary fiber; 1mg cholesterol; 418mg sodium.

Member Survey

Please answer the following questions to help your leader plan your First Place 4 Health meetings so that your needs might be met in this session. Give this form to your leader at the first group meeting.

Name _____   Birth date _____

Please list those who live in your household.

Name	Relationship	Age
_____	_____	_____
_____	_____	_____
_____	_____	_____
_____	_____	_____

What church do you attend? _____

Are you interested in receiving more information about our church?

      Yes   No

Occupation _____

What talent or area of expertise would you be willing to share with our class?

_____

Why did you join First Place 4 Health?

_____

With notice, would you be willing to lead a Bible study discussion one week?

      Yes   No

Are you comfortable praying out loud? _____

If the assistant leader were absent, would you be willing to assist in weighing in members and possibly evaluating the Live It Trackers?

      Yes   No

Any other comments:

_____

_____

Personal Weight and Measurement Record

Week	Weight	+ or -	Goal this Session	Pounds to goal
1				
2				
3				
4				
5				
6				
7				
8				
9				
10				
11				
12				

Beginning Measurements

Waist _____ Hips _____ Thighs _____ Chest _____

Ending Measurements

Waist _____ Hips _____ Thighs _____ Chest _____

First Place 4 Health
Prayer Partner

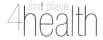

SCRIPTURE VERSE TO MEMORIZE FOR WEEK TWO:

Then Jesus declared, "I am the bread of life. He who comes to me will never go hungry, and he who believes in me will never be thirsty."

JOHN 6:35

Date: _____

Name: _____

Home Phone: ( ) _____

Work Phone: ( ) _____

Email: _____

Personal Prayer Concerns:

_____

_____

_____

_____

_____

_____

_____

This form is for prayer requests that are personal to you and your journey in First Place 4 Health. Please complete this form and have it ready to turn in when you arrive at your group meeting.

First Place 4 Health
Prayer Partner

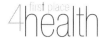

GOD'S BEST FOR
YOUR LIFE
Week
2

SCRIPTURE VERSE TO MEMORIZE FOR WEEK THREE:

"Ever since the time of your forefathers you have turned away from my decrees and have not kept them. Return to me, and I will return to you," says the LORD Almighty.

MALACHI 3:7

Date: _____

Name: _____

Home Phone: ( ) _____

Work Phone: ( ) _____

Email: _____

Personal Prayer Concerns:

_____

_____

_____

_____

_____

_____

_____

This form is for prayer requests that are personal to you and your journey in First Place 4 Health. Please complete this form and have it ready to turn in when you arrive at your group meeting.

First Place 4 Health
Prayer Partner

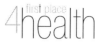

GOD'S BEST FOR
YOUR LIFE
Week
3

Date: _____

Name: _____

Home Phone: ( ) _____

Work Phone: ( ) _____

Email: _____

Personal Prayer Concerns:

_____

_____

_____

_____

_____

_____

_____

This form is for prayer requests that are personal to you and your journey in First Place 4 Health. Please complete this form and have it ready to turn in when you arrive at your group meeting.

First Place 4 Health
Prayer Partner

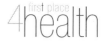

SCRIPTURE VERSE TO MEMORIZE FOR WEEK FIVE:

While we wait for the blessed hope—the glorious appearing of our great God and Savior, Jesus Christ, who gave himself for us to redeem us from all wickedness and to purify for himself a people that are his very own, eager to do what is good.

TITUS 2:13-14

Date: _____

Name: _____

Home Phone: (____) _____

Work Phone: (____) _____

Email: _____

Personal Prayer Concerns:

_____

_____

_____

_____

_____

_____

_____

This form is for prayer requests that are personal to you and your journey in First Place 4 Health. Please complete this form and have it ready to turn in when you arrive at your group meeting.

First Place 4 Health
Prayer Partner

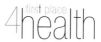

first place
4health

GOD'S BEST FOR
YOUR LIFE
Week
5

SCRIPTURE VERSE TO MEMORIZE FOR WEEK SIX:

The LORD does not look at the things man looks at. Man looks at the outward appearance, but the LORD looks at the heart.

1 SAMUEL 16:7

Date: _____

Name: _____

Home Phone: [_____] _____

Work Phone: [_____] _____

Email: _____

Personal Prayer Concerns:

_____

_____

_____

_____

_____

_____

_____

This form is for prayer requests that are personal to you and your journey in First Place 4 Health. Please complete this form and have it ready to turn in when you arrive at your group meeting.

First Place 4 Health
Prayer Partner

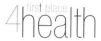

GOD'S BEST FOR
YOUR LIFE
Week
6

Date: _____

Name: _____

Home Phone: _____

Work Phone: _____

Email: _____

Personal Prayer Concerns:

_____

_____

_____

_____

_____

_____

_____

This form is for prayer requests that are personal to you and your journey in First Place 4 Health. Please complete this form and have it ready to turn in when you arrive at your group meeting.

First Place 4 Health
Prayer Partner

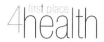

GOD'S BEST FOR
YOUR LIFE
Week
7

SCRIPTURE VERSE TO MEMORIZE FOR WEEK EIGHT:

My God will meet all your needs according to his glorious riches in Christ Jesus.

PHILIPPIANS 4:19

Date: _____

Name: _____

Home Phone: (____) _____

Work Phone: (____) _____

Email: _____

Personal Prayer Concerns:

_____

_____

_____

_____

_____

_____

_____

This form is for prayer requests that are personal to you and your journey in First Place 4 Health. Please complete this form and have it ready to turn in when you arrive at your group meeting.

First Place 4 Health
Prayer Partner

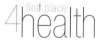

SCRIPTURE VERSE TO MEMORIZE FOR WEEK NINE:

Joshua told the people, "Consecrate yourselves, for tomorrow the LORD will do amazing things among you."

JOSHUA 3:5

Date: _____

Name: _____

Home Phone: _____

Work Phone: _____

Email: _____

Personal Prayer Concerns:

_____

_____

_____

_____

_____

_____

_____

This form is for prayer requests that are personal to you and your journey in First Place 4 Health. Please complete this form and have it ready to turn in when you arrive at your group meeting.

First Place 4 Health
Prayer Partner

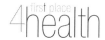

SCRIPTURE VERSE TO MEMORIZE FOR WEEK TEN:

My dear brothers, stand firm. Let nothing move you. Always give yourselves fully to the work of the Lord, because you know that your labor in the Lord is not in vain.

1 CORINTHIANS 15:58

Date: _____

Name: _____

Home Phone: (_____) _____

Work Phone: (_____) _____

Email: _____

Personal Prayer Concerns:

_____

_____

_____

_____

_____

_____

_____

This form is for prayer requests that are personal to you and your journey in First Place 4 Health. Please complete this form and have it ready to turn in when you arrive at your group meeting.

First Place 4 Health
Prayer Partner

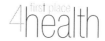

GOD'S BEST FOR
YOUR LIFE
Week
10

Date: _____

Name: _____

Home Phone: _____

Work Phone: _____

Email: _____

Personal Prayer Concerns:

_____

_____

_____

_____

_____

_____

_____

This form is for prayer requests that are personal to you and your journey in First Place 4 Health. Please complete this form and have it ready to turn in when you arrive at your group meeting.

First Place 4 Health
Prayer Partner

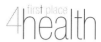

GOD'S BEST FOR
YOUR LIFE
Week
11

Date: ....

Name: _____

Home Phone: (_____) _____

Work Phone: (_____) _____

Email: _____

Personal Prayer Concerns:

_____

_____

_____

_____

_____

_____

_____

This form is for prayer requests that are personal to you and your journey in First Place 4 Health. Please complete this form and have it ready to turn in when you arrive at your group meeting.

Live It Tracker

Name: _____ Loss/gain: _____ lbs.

Date: _____ Week #: _____ Calorie Range: _____ My food goal for next week: _____

Activity Level: None, < 30 min/day, 30-60 min/day, 60+ min/day My activity goal for next week: _____

Group	Daily Calories							
	1300-1400	1500-1600	1700-1800	1900-2000	2100-2200	2300-2400	2500-2600	2700-2800
Fruits	1.5-2 c.	1.5-2 c.	1.5-2 c.	2-2.5 c.	2-2.5 c.	2.5-3.5 c.	3.5-4.5 c.	3.5-4.5 c.
Vegetables	1.5-2 c.	2-2.5 c.	2.5-3 c.	2.5-3 c.	3-3.5 c.	3.5-4.5 c.	4.5-5 c.	4.5-5 c.
Grains	5 oz-eq.	5-6 oz-eq.	6-7 oz-eq.	6-7 oz-eq.	7-8 oz-eq.	8-9 oz-eq.	9-10 oz-eq.	10-11 oz-eq.
Meat & Beans	4 oz-eq.	5 oz-eq.	5-5.5 oz-eq.	5.5-6.5 oz-eq.	6.5-7 oz-eq.	7-7.5 oz-eq.	7-7.5 oz-eq.	7.5-8 oz-eq.
Milk	2-3 c.	3 c.	3 c.	3 c.	3 c.	3 c.	3 c.	3 c.
Healthy Oils	4 tsp.	5 tsp.	5 tsp.	6 tsp.	6 tsp.	7 tsp.	8 tsp.	8 tsp.

Day/Date: ___

Breakfast: _____ Lunch: _____

Dinner: _____ Snack: _____

Group	Fruits	Vegetables	Grains	Meat & Beans	Milk	Oils
Goal Amount						
Estimate Your Total						
Increase ⇧ or Decrease? ⇩						

Physical Activity: _____ Spiritual Activity: _____

Steps/Miles/Minutes: _____

Day/Date: ___

Breakfast: _____ Lunch: _____

Dinner: _____ Snack: _____

Group	Fruits	Vegetables	Grains	Meat & Beans	Milk	Oils
Goal Amount						
Estimate Your Total						
Increase ⇧ or Decrease? ⇩						

Physical Activity: _____ Spiritual Activity: _____

Steps/Miles/Minutes: _____

Day/Date: ___

Breakfast: _____ Lunch: _____

Dinner: _____ Snack: _____

Group	Fruits	Vegetables	Grains	Meat & Beans	Milk	Oils
Goal Amount						
Estimate Your Total						
Increase ⇧ or Decrease? ⇩						

Physical Activity: _____ Spiritual Activity: _____

Steps/Miles/Minutes: _____

Day/Date:

Breakfast: _____   Lunch: _____

Dinner: _____   Snack: _____

Group	Fruits	Vegetables	Grains	Meat & Beans	Milk	Oils
Goal Amount						
Estimate Your Total						
Increase ⇧ or Decrease? ⇩						

Physical Activity: _____   Spiritual Activity: _____

Steps/Miles/Minutes: _____   _____

Day/Date:

Breakfast: _____   Lunch: _____

Dinner: _____   Snack: _____

Group	Fruits	Vegetables	Grains	Meat & Beans	Milk	Oils
Goal Amount						
Estimate Your Total						
Increase ⇧ or Decrease? ⇩						

Physical Activity: _____   Spiritual Activity: _____

Steps/Miles/Minutes: _____   _____

Day/Date:

Breakfast: _____   Lunch: _____

Dinner: _____   Snack: _____

Group	Fruits	Vegetables	Grains	Meat & Beans	Milk	Oils
Goal Amount						
Estimate Your Total						
Increase ⇧ or Decrease? ⇩						

Physical Activity: _____   Spiritual Activity: _____

Steps/Miles/Minutes: _____   _____

Day/Date:

Breakfast: _____   Lunch: _____

Dinner: _____   Snack: _____

Group	Fruits	Vegetables	Grains	Meat & Beans	Milk	Oils
Goal Amount						
Estimate Your Total						
Increase ⇧ or Decrease? ⇩						

Physical Activity: _____   Spiritual Activity: _____

Steps/Miles/Minutes: _____   _____

Live It Tracker

Name: _____ Loss/gain: _____ lbs.

Date: _____ Week #: _____ Calorie Range: _____ My food goal for next week: _____

Activity Level: None, < 30 min/day, 30-60 min/day, 60+ min/day My activity goal for next week: _____

Group	Daily Calories							
	1300-1400	1500-1600	1700-1800	1900-2000	2100-2200	2300-2400	2500-2600	2700-2800
Fruits	1.5-2 c.	1.5-2 c.	1.5-2 c.	2-2.5 c.	2-2.5 c.	2.5-3.5 c.	3.5-4.5 c.	3.5-4.5 c.
Vegetables	1.5-2 c.	2-2.5 c.	2.5-3 c.	2.5-3 c.	3-3.5 c.	3.5-4.5 c.	4.5-5 c.	4.5-5 c.
Grains	5 oz-eq.	5-6 oz-eq.	6-7 oz-eq.	6-7 oz-eq.	7-8 oz-eq.	8-9 oz-eq.	9-10 oz-eq.	10-11 oz-eq.
Meat & Beans	4 oz-eq.	5 oz-eq.	5-5.5 oz-eq.	5.5-6.5 oz-eq.	6.5-7 oz-eq.	7-7.5 oz-eq.	7-7.5 oz-eq.	7.5-8 oz-eq.
Milk	2-3 c.	3 c.	3 c.	3 c.	3 c.	3 c.	3 c.	3 c.
Healthy Oils	4 tsp.	5 tsp.	5 tsp.	6 tsp.	6 tsp.	7 tsp.	8 tsp.	8 tsp.

Day/Date:

Breakfast: _____   Lunch: _____

Dinner: _____   Snack: _____

Group	Fruits	Vegetables	Grains	Meat & Beans	Milk	Oils
Goal Amount						
Estimate Your Total						
Increase ⇧ or Decrease? ⇩						

Physical Activity: _____   Spiritual Activity: _____

Steps/Miles/Minutes: _____

Day/Date:

Breakfast: _____   Lunch: _____

Dinner: _____   Snack: _____

Group	Fruits	Vegetables	Grains	Meat & Beans	Milk	Oils
Goal Amount						
Estimate Your Total						
Increase ⇧ or Decrease? ⇩						

Physical Activity: _____   Spiritual Activity: _____

Steps/Miles/Minutes: _____

Day/Date:

Breakfast: _____   Lunch: _____

Dinner: _____   Snack: _____

Group	Fruits	Vegetables	Grains	Meat & Beans	Milk	Oils
Goal Amount						
Estimate Your Total						
Increase ⇧ or Decrease? ⇩						

Physical Activity: _____   Spiritual Activity: _____

Steps/Miles/Minutes: _____

Day/Date: _____

Breakfast: _____ Lunch: _____

Dinner: _____ Snack: _____

Group	Fruits	Vegetables	Grains	Meat & Beans	Milk	Oils
Goal Amount						
Estimate Your Total						
Increase ⇧ or Decrease? ⇩						

Physical Activity: _____ Spiritual Activity: _____

Steps/Miles/Minutes: _____ _____

Day/Date: _____

Breakfast: _____ Lunch: _____

Dinner: _____ Snack: _____

Group	Fruits	Vegetables	Grains	Meat & Beans	Milk	Oils
Goal Amount						
Estimate Your Total						
Increase ⇧ or Decrease? ⇩						

Physical Activity: _____ Spiritual Activity: _____

Steps/Miles/Minutes: _____ _____

Day/Date: _____

Breakfast: _____ Lunch: _____

Dinner: _____ Snack: _____

Group	Fruits	Vegetables	Grains	Meat & Beans	Milk	Oils
Goal Amount						
Estimate Your Total						
Increase ⇧ or Decrease? ⇩						

Physical Activity: _____ Spiritual Activity: _____

Steps/Miles/Minutes: _____ _____

Day/Date: _____

Breakfast: _____ Lunch: _____

Dinner: _____ Snack: _____

Group	Fruits	Vegetables	Grains	Meat & Beans	Milk	Oils
Goal Amount						
Estimate Your Total						
Increase ⇧ or Decrease? ⇩						

Physical Activity: _____ Spiritual Activity: _____

Steps/Miles/Minutes: _____ _____

Live It Tracker

Name: _____ Loss/gain: _____ lbs.

Date: _____ Week #: _____ Calorie Range: _____ My food goal for next week: _____

Activity Level: None, < 30 min/day, 30-60 min/day, 60+ min/day My activity goal for next week: _____

Group	Daily Calories							
	1300-1400	1500-1600	1700-1800	1900-2000	2100-2200	2300-2400	2500-2600	2700-2800
Fruits	1.5-2 c.	1.5-2 c.	1.5-2 c.	2-2.5 c.	2-2.5 c.	2.5-3.5 c.	3.5-4.5 c.	3.5-4.5 c.
Vegetables	1.5-2 c.	2-2.5 c.	2.5-3 c.	2.5-3 c.	3-3.5 c.	3.5-4.5 c.	4.5-5 c.	4.5-5 c.
Grains	5 oz-eq.	5-6 oz-eq.	6-7 oz-eq.	6-7 oz-eq.	7-8 oz-eq.	8-9 oz-eq.	9-10 oz-eq.	10-11 oz-eq.
Meat & Beans	4 oz-eq.	5 oz-eq.	5-5.5 oz-eq.	5.5-6.5 oz-eq.	6.5-7 oz-eq.	7-7.5 oz-eq.	7-7.5 oz-eq.	7.5-8 oz-eq.
Milk	2-3 c.	3 c.	3 c.	3 c.	3 c.	3 c.	3 c.	3 c.
Healthy Oils	4 tsp.	5 tsp.	5 tsp.	6 tsp.	6 tsp.	7 tsp.	8 tsp.	8 tsp.

Day/Date:

Breakfast: _____ Lunch: _____

Dinner: _____ Snack: _____

Group	Fruits	Vegetables	Grains	Meat & Beans	Milk	Oils
Goal Amount						
Estimate Your Total						
Increase ⇧ or Decrease? ⇩						

Physical Activity: _____ Spiritual Activity: _____

Steps/Miles/Minutes: _____

Day/Date:

Breakfast: _____ Lunch: _____

Dinner: _____ Snack: _____

Group	Fruits	Vegetables	Grains	Meat & Beans	Milk	Oils
Goal Amount						
Estimate Your Total						
Increase ⇧ or Decrease? ⇩						

Physical Activity: _____ Spiritual Activity: _____

Steps/Miles/Minutes: _____

Day/Date:

Breakfast: _____ Lunch: _____

Dinner: _____ Snack: _____

Group	Fruits	Vegetables	Grains	Meat & Beans	Milk	Oils
Goal Amount						
Estimate Your Total						
Increase ⇧ or Decrease? ⇩						

Physical Activity: _____ Spiritual Activity: _____

Steps/Miles/Minutes: _____

Day/Date: ___

Breakfast: _____ Lunch: _____

Dinner: _____ Snack: _____

Group	Fruits	Vegetables	Grains	Meat & Beans	Milk	Oils
Goal Amount						
Estimate Your Total						
Increase ⇧ or Decrease? ⇩						

Physical Activity: _____ Spiritual Activity: _____

Steps/Miles/Minutes: _____ _____

Day/Date: ___

Breakfast: _____ Lunch: _____

Dinner: _____ Snack: _____

Group	Fruits	Vegetables	Grains	Meat & Beans	Milk	Oils
Goal Amount						
Estimate Your Total						
Increase ⇧ or Decrease? ⇩						

Physical Activity: _____ Spiritual Activity: _____

Steps/Miles/Minutes: _____ _____

Day/Date: ___

Breakfast: _____ Lunch: _____

Dinner: _____ Snack: _____

Group	Fruits	Vegetables	Grains	Meat & Beans	Milk	Oils
Goal Amount						
Estimate Your Total						
Increase ⇧ or Decrease? ⇩						

Physical Activity: _____ Spiritual Activity: _____

Steps/Miles/Minutes: _____ _____

Day/Date: ___

Breakfast: _____ Lunch: _____

Dinner: _____ Snack: _____

Group	Fruits	Vegetables	Grains	Meat & Beans	Milk	Oils
Goal Amount						
Estimate Your Total						
Increase ⇧ or Decrease? ⇩						

Physical Activity: _____ Spiritual Activity: _____

Steps/Miles/Minutes: _____ _____

Live It Tracker

Name: _____ Loss/gain: _____ lbs.

Date: _____ Week #: _____ Calorie Range: _____ My food goal for next week: _____

Activity Level: None, < 30 min/day, 30-60 min/day, 60+ min/day My activity goal for next week: _____

Group	Daily Calories							
	1300-1400	1500-1600	1700-1800	1900-2000	2100-2200	2300-2400	2500-2600	2700-2800
Fruits	1.5-2 c.	1.5-2 c.	1.5-2 c.	2-2.5 c.	2-2.5 c.	2.5-3.5 c.	3.5-4.5 c.	3.5-4.5 c.
Vegetables	1.5-2 c.	2-2.5 c.	2.5-3 c.	2.5-3 c.	3-3.5 c.	3.5-4.5 c.	4.5-5 c.	4.5-5 c.
Grains	5 oz-eq.	5-6 oz-eq.	6-7 oz-eq.	6-7 oz-eq.	7-8 oz-eq.	8-9 oz-eq.	9-10 oz-eq.	10-11 oz-eq.
Meat & Beans	4 oz-eq.	5 oz-eq.	5-5.5 oz-eq.	5.5-6.5 oz-eq.	6.5-7 oz-eq.	7-7.5 oz-eq.	7-7.5 oz-eq.	7.5-8 oz-eq.
Milk	2-3 c.	3 c.	3 c.	3 c.	3 c.	3 c.	3 c.	3 c.
Healthy Oils	4 tsp.	5 tsp.	5 tsp.	6 tsp.	6 tsp.	7 tsp.	8 tsp.	8 tsp.

Day/Date:

Breakfast: _____ Lunch: _____

Dinner: _____ Snack: _____

Group	Fruits	Vegetables	Grains	Meat & Beans	Milk	Oils
Goal Amount						
Estimate Your Total						
Increase ⇧ or Decrease? ⇩						

Physical Activity: _____ Spiritual Activity: _____

Steps/Miles/Minutes: _____

Day/Date:

Breakfast: _____ Lunch: _____

Dinner: _____ Snack: _____

Group	Fruits	Vegetables	Grains	Meat & Beans	Milk	Oils
Goal Amount						
Estimate Your Total						
Increase ⇧ or Decrease? ⇩						

Physical Activity: _____ Spiritual Activity: _____

Steps/Miles/Minutes: _____

Day/Date:

Breakfast: _____ Lunch: _____

Dinner: _____ Snack: _____

Group	Fruits	Vegetables	Grains	Meat & Beans	Milk	Oils
Goal Amount						
Estimate Your Total						
Increase ⇧ or Decrease? ⇩						

Physical Activity: _____ Spiritual Activity: _____

Steps/Miles/Minutes: _____

Day/Date:

Breakfast: _____ Lunch: _____

Dinner: _____ Snack: _____

Group	Fruits	Vegetables	Grains	Meat & Beans	Milk	Oils
Goal Amount						
Estimate Your Total						
Increase ⇧ or Decrease? ⇩						

Physical Activity: _____ Spiritual Activity: _____

Steps/Miles/Minutes: _____ _____

Day/Date:

Breakfast: _____ Lunch: _____

Dinner: _____ Snack: _____

Group	Fruits	Vegetables	Grains	Meat & Beans	Milk	Oils
Goal Amount						
Estimate Your Total						
Increase ⇧ or Decrease? ⇩						

Physical Activity: _____ Spiritual Activity: _____

Steps/Miles/Minutes: _____ _____

Day/Date:

Breakfast: _____ Lunch: _____

Dinner: _____ Snack: _____

Group	Fruits	Vegetables	Grains	Meat & Beans	Milk	Oils
Goal Amount						
Estimate Your Total						
Increase ⇧ or Decrease? ⇩						

Physical Activity: _____ Spiritual Activity: _____

Steps/Miles/Minutes: _____ _____

Day/Date:

Breakfast: _____ Lunch: _____

Dinner: _____ Snack: _____

Group	Fruits	Vegetables	Grains	Meat & Beans	Milk	Oils
Goal Amount						
Estimate Your Total						
Increase ⇧ or Decrease? ⇩						

Physical Activity: _____ Spiritual Activity: _____

Steps/Miles/Minutes: _____ _____

Live It Tracker

Name: _____ Loss/gain: _____ lbs.

Date: _____ Week #: _____ Calorie Range: _____ My food goal for next week: _____

Activity Level: None, < 30 min/day, 30-60 min/day, 60+ min/day My activity goal for next week: _____

Group	Daily Calories							
	1300-1400	1500-1600	1700-1800	1900-2000	2100-2200	2300-2400	2500-2600	2700-2800
Fruits	1.5-2 c.	1.5-2 c.	1.5-2 c.	2-2.5 c.	2-2.5 c.	2.5-3.5 c.	3.5-4.5 c.	3.5-4.5 c.
Vegetables	1.5-2 c.	2-2.5 c.	2.5-3 c.	2.5-3 c.	3-3.5 c.	3.5-4.5 c.	4.5-5 c.	4.5-5 c.
Grains	5 oz-eq.	5-6 oz-eq.	6-7 oz-eq.	6-7 oz-eq.	7-8 oz-eq.	8-9 oz-eq.	9-10 oz-eq.	10-11 oz-eq.
Meat & Beans	4 oz-eq.	5 oz-eq.	5-5.5 oz-eq.	5.5-6.5 oz-eq.	6.5-7 oz-eq.	7-7.5 oz-eq.	7-7.5 oz-eq.	7.5-8 oz-eq.
Milk	2-3 c.	3 c.	3 c.	3 c.	3 c.	3 c.	3 c.	3 c.
Healthy Oils	4 tsp.	5 tsp.	5 tsp.	6 tsp.	6 tsp.	7 tsp.	8 tsp.	8 tsp.

Day/Date: _____

Breakfast: _____ Lunch: _____

Dinner: _____ Snack: _____

Group	Fruits	Vegetables	Grains	Meat & Beans	Milk	Oils
Goal Amount						
Estimate Your Total						
Increase ⇧ or Decrease? ⇩						

Physical Activity: _____ Spiritual Activity: _____

Steps/Miles/Minutes: _____ _____

Day/Date: _____

Breakfast: _____ Lunch: _____

Dinner: _____ Snack: _____

Group	Fruits	Vegetables	Grains	Meat & Beans	Milk	Oils
Goal Amount						
Estimate Your Total						
Increase ⇧ or Decrease? ⇩						

Physical Activity: _____ Spiritual Activity: _____

Steps/Miles/Minutes: _____ _____

Day/Date: _____

Breakfast: _____ Lunch: _____

Dinner: _____ Snack: _____

Group	Fruits	Vegetables	Grains	Meat & Beans	Milk	Oils
Goal Amount						
Estimate Your Total						
Increase ⇧ or Decrease? ⇩						

Physical Activity: _____ Spiritual Activity: _____

Steps/Miles/Minutes: _____

Day/Date:

Breakfast: _____   Lunch: _____

Dinner: _____   Snack: _____

Group	Fruits	Vegetables	Grains	Meat & Beans	Milk	Oils
Goal Amount						
Estimate Your Total						
Increase ⇧ or Decrease? ⇩						

Physical Activity: _____   Spiritual Activity: _____

Steps/Miles/Minutes: _____   _____

Day/Date:

Breakfast: _____   Lunch: _____

Dinner: _____   Snack: _____

Group	Fruits	Vegetables	Grains	Meat & Beans	Milk	Oils
Goal Amount						
Estimate Your Total						
Increase ⇧ or Decrease? ⇩						

Physical Activity: _____   Spiritual Activity: _____

Steps/Miles/Minutes: _____   _____

Day/Date:

Breakfast: _____   Lunch: _____

Dinner: _____   Snack: _____

Group	Fruits	Vegetables	Grains	Meat & Beans	Milk	Oils
Goal Amount						
Estimate Your Total						
Increase ⇧ or Decrease? ⇩						

Physical Activity: _____   Spiritual Activity: _____

Steps/Miles/Minutes: _____   _____

Day/Date:

Breakfast: _____   Lunch: _____

Dinner: _____   Snack: _____

Group	Fruits	Vegetables	Grains	Meat & Beans	Milk	Oils
Goal Amount						
Estimate Your Total						
Increase ⇧ or Decrease? ⇩						

Physical Activity: _____   Spiritual Activity: _____

Steps/Miles/Minutes: _____   _____

Live It Tracker

Name: _____ Loss/gain: _____ lbs.

Date: _____ Week #: ____ Calorie Range: _____ My food goal for next week: _____

Activity Level: None, < 30 min/day, 30-60 min/day, 60+ min/day My activity goal for next week: _____

Group	Daily Calories							
	1300-1400	1500-1600	1700-1800	1900-2000	2100-2200	2300-2400	2500-2600	2700-2800
Fruits	1.5-2 c.	1.5-2 c.	1.5-2 c.	2-2.5 c.	2-2.5 c.	2.5-3.5 c.	3.5-4.5 c.	3.5-4.5 c.
Vegetables	1.5-2 c.	2-2.5 c.	2.5-3 c.	2.5-3 c.	3-3.5 c.	3.5-4.5 c.	4.5-5 c.	4.5-5 c.
Grains	5 oz-eq.	5-6 oz-eq.	6-7 oz-eq.	6-7 oz-eq.	7-8 oz-eq.	8-9 oz-eq.	9-10 oz-eq.	10-11 oz-eq.
Meat & Beans	4 oz-eq.	5 oz-eq.	5-5.5 oz-eq.	5.5-6.5 oz-eq.	6.5-7 oz-eq.	7-7.5 oz-eq.	7-7.5 oz-eq.	7.5-8 oz-eq.
Milk	2-3 c.	3 c.	3 c.	3 c.	3 c.	3 c.	3 c.	3 c.
Healthy Oils	4 tsp.	5 tsp.	5 tsp.	6 tsp.	6 tsp.	7 tsp.	8 tsp.	8 tsp.

Day/Date:

Breakfast: _____ Lunch: _____

Dinner: _____ Snack: _____

Group	Fruits	Vegetables	Grains	Meat & Beans	Milk	Oils
Goal Amount						
Estimate Your Total						
Increase ⇧ or Decrease? ⇩						

Physical Activity: _____ Spiritual Activity: _____

Steps/Miles/Minutes: _____

Day/Date:

Breakfast: _____ Lunch: _____

Dinner: _____ Snack: _____

Group	Fruits	Vegetables	Grains	Meat & Beans	Milk	Oils
Goal Amount						
Estimate Your Total						
Increase ⇧ or Decrease? ⇩						

Physical Activity: _____ Spiritual Activity: _____

Steps/Miles/Minutes: _____

Day/Date:

Breakfast: _____ Lunch: _____

Dinner: _____ Snack: _____

Group	Fruits	Vegetables	Grains	Meat & Beans	Milk	Oils
Goal Amount						
Estimate Your Total						
Increase ⇧ or Decrease? ⇩						

Physical Activity: _____ Spiritual Activity: _____

Steps/Miles/Minutes: _____

Day/Date:

Breakfast: _____   Lunch: _____

Dinner: _____   Snack: _____

Group	Fruits	Vegetables	Grains	Meat & Beans	Milk	Oils
Goal Amount						
Estimate Your Total						
Increase ⬆ or Decrease? ⬇						

Physical Activity: _____   Spiritual Activity: _____

Steps/Miles/Minutes: _____   _____

Day/Date:

Breakfast: _____   Lunch: _____

Dinner: _____   Snack: _____

Group	Fruits	Vegetables	Grains	Meat & Beans	Milk	Oils
Goal Amount						
Estimate Your Total						
Increase ⬆ or Decrease? ⬇						

Physical Activity: _____   Spiritual Activity: _____

Steps/Miles/Minutes: _____   _____

Day/Date:

Breakfast: _____   Lunch: _____

Dinner: _____   Snack: _____

Group	Fruits	Vegetables	Grains	Meat & Beans	Milk	Oils
Goal Amount						
Estimate Your Total						
Increase ⬆ or Decrease? ⬇						

Physical Activity: _____   Spiritual Activity: _____

Steps/Miles/Minutes: _____   _____

Day/Date:

Breakfast: _____   Lunch: _____

Dinner: _____   Snack: _____

Group	Fruits	Vegetables	Grains	Meat & Beans	Milk	Oils
Goal Amount						
Estimate Your Total						
Increase ⬆ or Decrease? ⬇						

Physical Activity: _____   Spiritual Activity: _____

Steps/Miles/Minutes: _____   _____

Live It Tracker

Name: _____ Loss/gain: _____ lbs.

Date: _____ Week #: _____ Calorie Range: _____ My food goal for next week: _____

Activity Level: None, < 30 min/day, 30-60 min/day, 60+ min/day My activity goal for next week: _____

Group	Daily Calories							
	1300-1400	1500-1600	1700-1800	1900-2000	2100-2200	2300-2400	2500-2600	2700-2800
Fruits	1.5-2 c.	1.5-2 c.	1.5-2 c.	2-2.5 c.	2-2.5 c.	2.5-3.5 c.	3.5-4.5 c.	3.5-4.5 c.
Vegetables	1.5-2 c.	2-2.5 c.	2.5-3 c.	2.5-3 c.	3-3.5 c.	3.5-4.5 c.	4.5-5 c.	4.5-5 c.
Grains	5 oz-eq.	5-6 oz-eq.	6-7 oz-eq.	6-7 oz-eq.	7-8 oz-eq.	8-9 oz-eq.	9-10 oz-eq.	10-11 oz-eq.
Meat & Beans	4 oz-eq.	5 oz-eq.	5-5.5 oz-eq.	5.5-6.5 oz-eq.	6.5-7 oz-eq.	7-7.5 oz-eq.	7-7.5 oz-eq.	7.5-8 oz-eq.
Milk	2-3 c.	3 c.	3 c.	3 c.	3 c.	3 c.	3 c.	3 c.
Healthy Oils	4 tsp.	5 tsp.	5 tsp.	6 tsp.	6 tsp.	7 tsp.	8 tsp.	8 tsp.

Day/Date:

Breakfast: _____ Lunch: _____

Dinner: _____ Snack: _____

Group	Fruits	Vegetables	Grains	Meat & Beans	Milk	Oils
Goal Amount						
Estimate Your Total						
Increase ⬆ or Decrease? ⬇						

Physical Activity: _____ Spiritual Activity: _____

Steps/Miles/Minutes: _____

Day/Date:

Breakfast: _____ Lunch: _____

Dinner: _____ Snack: _____

Group	Fruits	Vegetables	Grains	Meat & Beans	Milk	Oils
Goal Amount						
Estimate Your Total						
Increase ⬆ or Decrease? ⬇						

Physical Activity: _____ Spiritual Activity: _____

Steps/Miles/Minutes: _____

Day/Date:

Breakfast: _____ Lunch: _____

Dinner: _____ Snack: _____

Group	Fruits	Vegetables	Grains	Meat & Beans	Milk	Oils
Goal Amount						
Estimate Your Total						
Increase ⬆ or Decrease? ⬇						

Physical Activity: _____ Spiritual Activity: _____

Steps/Miles/Minutes: _____

Day/Date:

Breakfast: _____   Lunch: _____

Dinner: _____   Snack: _____

Group	Fruits	Vegetables	Grains	Meat & Beans	Milk	Oils
Goal Amount						
Estimate Your Total						
Increase ⬆ or Decrease? ⬇						

Physical Activity: _____   Spiritual Activity: _____

Steps/Miles/Minutes: _____   _____

Day/Date:

Breakfast: _____   Lunch: _____

Dinner: _____   Snack: _____

Group	Fruits	Vegetables	Grains	Meat & Beans	Milk	Oils
Goal Amount						
Estimate Your Total						
Increase ⬆ or Decrease? ⬇						

Physical Activity: _____   Spiritual Activity: _____

Steps/Miles/Minutes: _____   _____

Day/Date:

Breakfast: _____   Lunch: _____

Dinner: _____   Snack: _____

Group	Fruits	Vegetables	Grains	Meat & Beans	Milk	Oils
Goal Amount						
Estimate Your Total						
Increase ⬆ or Decrease? ⬇						

Physical Activity: _____   Spiritual Activity: _____

Steps/Miles/Minutes: _____   _____

Day/Date:

Breakfast: _____   Lunch: _____

Dinner: _____   Snack: _____

Group	Fruits	Vegetables	Grains	Meat & Beans	Milk	Oils
Goal Amount						
Estimate Your Total						
Increase ⬆ or Decrease? ⬇						

Physical Activity: _____   Spiritual Activity: _____

Steps/Miles/Minutes: _____   _____

Live It Tracker

Name: _____ Loss/gain: _____ lbs.

Date: _____ Week #: ____ Calorie Range: _____ My food goal for next week: _____

Activity Level: None, < 30 min/day, 30-60 min/day, 60+ min/day My activity goal for next week: _____

Group	Daily Calories							
	1300-1400	1500-1600	1700-1800	1900-2000	2100-2200	2300-2400	2500-2600	2700-2800
Fruits	1.5-2 c.	1.5-2 c.	1.5-2 c.	2-2.5 c.	2-2.5 c.	2.5-3.5 c.	3.5-4.5 c.	3.5-4.5 c.
Vegetables	1.5-2 c.	2-2.5 c.	2.5-3 c.	2.5-3 c.	3-3.5 c.	3.5-4.5 c.	4.5-5 c.	4.5-5 c.
Grains	5 oz-eq.	5-6 oz-eq.	6-7 oz-eq.	6-7 oz-eq.	7-8 oz-eq.	8-9 oz-eq.	9-10 oz-eq.	10-11 oz-eq.
Meat & Beans	4 oz-eq.	5 oz-eq.	5-5.5 oz-eq.	5.5-6.5 oz-eq.	6.5-7 oz-eq.	7-7.5 oz-eq.	7-7.5 oz-eq.	7.5-8 oz-eq.
Milk	2-3 c.	3 c.	3 c.	3 c.	3 c.	3 c.	3 c.	3 c.
Healthy Oils	4 tsp.	5 tsp.	5 tsp.	6 tsp.	6 tsp.	7 tsp.	8 tsp.	8 tsp.

Day/Date: _____

Breakfast: _____ Lunch: _____

Dinner: _____ Snack: _____

Group	Fruits	Vegetables	Grains	Meat & Beans	Milk	Oils
Goal Amount						
Estimate Your Total						
Increase ⇧ or Decrease? ⇩						

Physical Activity: _____ Spiritual Activity: _____

Steps/Miles/Minutes: _____ _____

Day/Date: _____

Breakfast: _____ Lunch: _____

Dinner: _____ Snack: _____

Group	Fruits	Vegetables	Grains	Meat & Beans	Milk	Oils
Goal Amount						
Estimate Your Total						
Increase ⇧ or Decrease? ⇩						

Physical Activity: _____ Spiritual Activity: _____

Steps/Miles/Minutes: _____ _____

Day/Date: _____

Breakfast: _____ Lunch: _____

Dinner: _____ Snack: _____

Group	Fruits	Vegetables	Grains	Meat & Beans	Milk	Oils
Goal Amount						
Estimate Your Total						
Increase ⇧ or Decrease? ⇩						

Physical Activity: _____ Spiritual Activity: _____

Steps/Miles/Minutes: _____ _____

Day/Date: _____

Breakfast: _____ Lunch: _____

Dinner: _____ Snack: _____

Group	Fruits	Vegetables	Grains	Meat & Beans	Milk	Oils
Goal Amount						
Estimate Your Total						
Increase ⇧ or Decrease? ⇩						

Physical Activity: _____ Spiritual Activity: _____

Steps/Miles/Minutes: _____ _____

Day/Date: _____

Breakfast: _____ Lunch: _____

Dinner: _____ Snack: _____

Group	Fruits	Vegetables	Grains	Meat & Beans	Milk	Oils
Goal Amount						
Estimate Your Total						
Increase ⇧ or Decrease? ⇩						

Physical Activity: _____ Spiritual Activity: _____

Steps/Miles/Minutes: _____ _____

Day/Date: _____

Breakfast: _____ Lunch: _____

Dinner: _____ Snack: _____

Group	Fruits	Vegetables	Grains	Meat & Beans	Milk	Oils
Goal Amount						
Estimate Your Total						
Increase ⇧ or Decrease? ⇩						

Physical Activity: _____ Spiritual Activity: _____

Steps/Miles/Minutes: _____ _____

Day/Date: _____

Breakfast: _____ Lunch: _____

Dinner: _____ Snack: _____

Group	Fruits	Vegetables	Grains	Meat & Beans	Milk	Oils
Goal Amount						
Estimate Your Total						
Increase ⇧ or Decrease? ⇩						

Physical Activity: _____ Spiritual Activity: _____

Steps/Miles/Minutes: _____ _____

Live It Tracker

Name: _____ Loss/gain: _____ lbs.

Date: _____ Week #: _____ Calorie Range: _____ My food goal for next week: _____

Activity Level: None, < 30 min/day, 30-60 min/day, 60+ min/day My activity goal for next week: _____

Group	Daily Calories							
	1300-1400	1500-1600	1700-1800	1900-2000	2100-2200	2300-2400	2500-2600	2700-2800
Fruits	1.5-2 c.	1.5-2 c.	1.5-2 c.	2-2.5 c.	2-2.5 c.	2.5-3.5 c.	3.5-4.5 c.	3.5-4.5 c.
Vegetables	1.5-2 c.	2-2.5 c.	2.5-3 c.	2.5-3 c.	3-3.5 c.	3.5-4.5 c.	4.5-5 c.	4.5-5 c.
Grains	5 oz-eq.	5-6 oz-eq.	6-7 oz-eq.	6-7 oz-eq.	7-8 oz-eq.	8-9 oz-eq.	9-10 oz-eq.	10-11 oz-eq.
Meat & Beans	4 oz-eq.	5 oz-eq.	5-5.5 oz-eq.	5.5-6.5 oz-eq.	6.5-7 oz-eq.	7-7.5 oz-eq.	7-7.5 oz-eq.	7.5-8 oz-eq.
Milk	2-3 c.	3 c.	3 c.	3 c.	3 c.	3 c.	3 c.	3 c.
Healthy Oils	4 tsp.	5 tsp.	5 tsp.	6 tsp.	6 tsp.	7 tsp.	8 tsp.	8 tsp.

Day/Date: _____

Breakfast: _____ Lunch: _____

Dinner: _____ Snack: _____

Group	Fruits	Vegetables	Grains	Meat & Beans	Milk	Oils
Goal Amount						
Estimate Your Total						
Increase ⇧ or Decrease? ⇩						

Physical Activity: _____ Spiritual Activity: _____

Steps/Miles/Minutes: _____

Day/Date: _____

Breakfast: _____ Lunch: _____

Dinner: _____ Snack: _____

Group	Fruits	Vegetables	Grains	Meat & Beans	Milk	Oils
Goal Amount						
Estimate Your Total						
Increase ⇧ or Decrease? ⇩						

Physical Activity: _____ Spiritual Activity: _____

Steps/Miles/Minutes: _____

Day/Date: _____

Breakfast: _____ Lunch: _____

Dinner: _____ Snack: _____

Group	Fruits	Vegetables	Grains	Meat & Beans	Milk	Oils
Goal Amount						
Estimate Your Total						
Increase ⇧ or Decrease? ⇩						

Physical Activity: _____ Spiritual Activity: _____

Steps/Miles/Minutes: _____

Day/Date: _____

Breakfast: _____ Lunch: _____

Dinner: _____ Snack: _____

Group	Fruits	Vegetables	Grains	Meat & Beans	Milk	Oils
Goal Amount						
Estimate Your Total						
Increase ⬆ or Decrease? ⬇						

Physical Activity: _____ Spiritual Activity: _____

Steps/Miles/Minutes: _____ _____

Day/Date: _____

Breakfast: _____ Lunch: _____

Dinner: _____ Snack: _____

Group	Fruits	Vegetables	Grains	Meat & Beans	Milk	Oils
Goal Amount						
Estimate Your Total						
Increase ⬆ or Decrease? ⬇						

Physical Activity: _____ Spiritual Activity: _____

Steps/Miles/Minutes: _____ _____

Day/Date: _____

Breakfast: _____ Lunch: _____

Dinner: _____ Snack: _____

Group	Fruits	Vegetables	Grains	Meat & Beans	Milk	Oils
Goal Amount						
Estimate Your Total						
Increase ⬆ or Decrease? ⬇						

Physical Activity: _____ Spiritual Activity: _____

Steps/Miles/Minutes: _____ _____

Day/Date: _____

Breakfast: _____ Lunch: _____

Dinner: _____ Snack: _____

Group	Fruits	Vegetables	Grains	Meat & Beans	Milk	Oils
Goal Amount						
Estimate Your Total						
Increase ⬆ or Decrease? ⬇						

Physical Activity: _____ Spiritual Activity: _____

Steps/Miles/Minutes: _____ _____

Live It Tracker

Name: _____ Loss/gain: _____ lbs.

Date: _____ Week #: _____ Calorie Range: _____ My food goal for next week: _____

Activity Level: None, < 30 min/day, 30-60 min/day, 60+ min/day My activity goal for next week: _____

Group	Daily Calories							
	1300-1400	1500-1600	1700-1800	1900-2000	2100-2200	2300-2400	2500-2600	2700-2800
Fruits	1.5-2 c.	1.5-2 c.	1.5-2 c.	2-2.5 c.	2-2.5 c.	2.5-3.5 c.	3.5-4.5 c.	3.5-4.5 c.
Vegetables	1.5-2 c.	2-2.5 c.	2.5-3 c.	2.5-3 c.	3-3.5 c.	3.5-4.5 c.	4.5-5 c.	4.5-5 c.
Grains	5 oz-eq.	5-6 oz-eq.	6-7 oz-eq.	6-7 oz-eq.	7-8 oz-eq.	8-9 oz-eq.	9-10 oz-eq.	10-11 oz-eq.
Meat & Beans	4 oz-eq.	5 oz eq.	5-5.5 oz-eq.	5.5-6.5 oz-eq.	6.5-7 oz-eq.	7-7.5 oz-eq.	7-7.5 oz-eq.	7.5-8 oz-eq.
Milk	2-3 c.	3 c.	3 c.	3 c.	3 c.	3 c.	3 c.	3 c.
Healthy Oils	4 tsp.	5 tsp.	5 tsp.	6 tsp.	6 tsp.	7 tsp.	8 tsp.	8 tsp.

Day/Date: _____

Breakfast: _____ Lunch: _____

Dinner: _____ Snack: _____

Group	Fruits	Vegetables	Grains	Meat & Beans	Milk	Oils
Goal Amount						
Estimate Your Total						
Increase ⇧ or Decrease? ⇩						

Physical Activity: _____ Spiritual Activity: _____

Steps/Miles/Minutes: _____

Day/Date: _____

Breakfast: _____ Lunch: _____

Dinner: _____ Snack: _____

Group	Fruits	Vegetables	Grains	Meat & Beans	Milk	Oils
Goal Amount						
Estimate Your Total						
Increase ⇧ or Decrease? ⇩						

Physical Activity: _____ Spiritual Activity: _____

Steps/Miles/Minutes: _____

Day/Date: _____

Breakfast: _____ Lunch: _____

Dinner: _____ Snack: _____

Group	Fruits	Vegetables	Grains	Meat & Beans	Milk	Oils
Goal Amount						
Estimate Your Total						
Increase ⇧ or Decrease? ⇩						

Physical Activity: _____ Spiritual Activity: _____

Steps/Miles/Minutes: _____

Breakfast: _____   **Lunch:** _____

Dinner: _____   **Snack:** _____

Group	Fruits	Vegetables	Grains	Meat & Beans	Milk	Oils
Goal Amount						
Estimate Your Total						
Increase ⇧ or Decrease? ⇩						

Physical Activity: _____   **Spiritual Activity:** _____

Steps/Miles/Minutes: _____

Day/Date:

Breakfast: _____   **Lunch:** _____

Dinner: _____   **Snack:** _____

Group	Fruits	Vegetables	Grains	Meat & Beans	Milk	Oils
Goal Amount						
Estimate Your Total						
Increase ⇧ or Decrease? ⇩						

Physical Activity: _____   **Spiritual Activity:** _____

Steps/Miles/Minutes: _____

Day/Date:

Breakfast: _____   **Lunch:** _____

Dinner: _____   **Snack:** _____

Group	Fruits	Vegetables	Grains	Meat & Beans	Milk	Oils
Goal Amount						
Estimate Your Total						
Increase ⇧ or Decrease? ⇩						

Physical Activity: _____   **Spiritual Activity:** _____

Steps/Miles/Minutes: _____

Day/Date:

Breakfast: _____   **Lunch:** _____

Dinner: _____   **Snack:** _____

Group	Fruits	Vegetables	Grains	Meat & Beans	Milk	Oils
Goal Amount						
Estimate Your Total						
Increase ⇧ or Decrease? ⇩						

Physical Activity: _____   **Spiritual Activity:** _____

Steps/Miles/Minutes: _____

Day/Date:

Live It Tracker

Name: _____ Loss/gain: _____ lbs.

Date: _____ Week #: _____ Calorie Range: _____ My food goal for next week: _____

Activity Level: None, < 30 min/day, 30-60 min/day, 60+ min/day My activity goal for next week: _____

Group	Daily Calories							
	1300-1400	1500-1600	1700-1800	1900-2000	2100-2200	2300-2400	2500-2600	2700-2800
Fruits	1.5-2 c.	1.5-2 c.	1.5-2 c.	2-2.5 c.	2-2.5 c.	2.5-3.5 c.	3.5-4.5 c.	3.5-4.5 c.
Vegetables	1.5-2 c.	2-2.5 c.	2.5-3 c.	2.5-3 c.	3-3.5 c.	3.5-4.5 c.	4.5-5 c.	4.5-5 c.
Grains	5 oz-eq.	5-6 oz-eq.	6-7 oz-eq.	6-7 oz-eq.	7-8 oz-eq.	8-9 oz-eq.	9-10 oz-eq.	10-11 oz-eq.
Meat & Beans	4 oz-eq.	5 oz-eq.	5-5.5 oz-eq.	5.5-6.5 oz-eq.	6.5-7 oz-eq.	7-7.5 oz-eq.	7-7.5 oz-eq.	7.5-8 oz-eq.
Milk	2-3 c.	3 c.	3 c.	3 c.	3 c.	3 c.	3 c.	3 c.
Healthy Oils	4 tsp.	5 tsp.	5 tsp.	6 tsp.	6 tsp.	7 tsp.	8 tsp.	8 tsp.

Day/Date: _____

Breakfast: _____ Lunch: _____

Dinner: _____ Snack: _____

Group	Fruits	Vegetables	Grains	Meat & Beans	Milk	Oils
Goal Amount						
Estimate Your Total						
Increase ⇧ or Decrease? ⇩						

Physical Activity: _____ Spiritual Activity: _____

Steps/Miles/Minutes: _____

Day/Date: _____

Breakfast: _____ Lunch: _____

Dinner: _____ Snack: _____

Group	Fruits	Vegetables	Grains	Meat & Beans	Milk	Oils
Goal Amount						
Estimate Your Total						
Increase ⇧ or Decrease? ⇩						

Physical Activity: _____ Spiritual Activity: _____

Steps/Miles/Minutes: _____

Day/Date: _____

Breakfast: _____ Lunch: _____

Dinner: _____ Snack: _____

Group	Fruits	Vegetables	Grains	Meat & Beans	Milk	Oils
Goal Amount						
Estimate Your Total						
Increase ⇧ or Decrease? ⇩						

Physical Activity: _____ Spiritual Activity: _____

Steps/Miles/Minutes: _____

Day/Date: _____

Breakfast: _____ Lunch: _____

Dinner: _____ Snack: _____

Group	Fruits	Vegetables	Grains	Meat & Beans	Milk	Oils
Goal Amount						
Estimate Your Total						
Increase ⬆ or Decrease? ⬇						

Physical Activity: _____ Spiritual Activity: _____

Steps/Miles/Minutes: _____ _____

Day/Date: _____

Breakfast: _____ Lunch: _____

Dinner: _____ Snack: _____

Group	Fruits	Vegetables	Grains	Meat & Beans	Milk	Oils
Goal Amount						
Estimate Your Total						
Increase ⬆ or Decrease? ⬇						

Physical Activity: _____ Spiritual Activity: _____

Steps/Miles/Minutes: _____ _____

Day/Date: _____

Breakfast: _____ Lunch: _____

Dinner: _____ Snack: _____

Group	Fruits	Vegetables	Grains	Meat & Beans	Milk	Oils
Goal Amount						
Estimate Your Total						
Increase ⬆ or Decrease? ⬇						

Physical Activity: _____ Spiritual Activity: _____

Steps/Miles/Minutes: _____ _____

Day/Date: _____

Breakfast: _____ Lunch: _____

Dinner: _____ Snack: _____

Group	Fruits	Vegetables	Grains	Meat & Beans	Milk	Oils
Goal Amount						
Estimate Your Total						
Increase ⬆ or Decrease? ⬇						

Physical Activity: _____ Spiritual Activity: _____

Steps/Miles/Minutes: _____ _____

Live It Tracker

Name: _____ Loss/gain: _____ lbs.

Date: _____ Week #: _____ Calorie Range: _____ My food goal for next week: _____

Activity Level: None, < 30 min/day, 30-60 min/day, 60+ min/day My activity goal for next week: _____

Group	Daily Calories							
	1300-1400	1500-1600	1700-1800	1900-2000	2100-2200	2300-2400	2500-2600	2700-2800
Fruits	1.5-2 c.	1.5-2 c.	1.5-2 c.	2-2.5 c.	2-2.5 c.	2.5-3.5 c.	3.5-4.5 c.	3.5-4.5 c.
Vegetables	1.5-2 c.	2-2.5 c.	2.5-3 c.	2.5-3 c.	3-3.5 c.	3.5-4.5 c.	4.5-5 c.	4.5-5 c.
Grains	5 oz-eq.	5-6 oz-eq.	6-7 oz-eq.	6-7 oz-eq.	7-8 oz-eq.	8-9 oz-eq.	9-10 oz-eq.	10-11 oz-eq.
Meat & Beans	4 oz-eq.	5 oz-eq.	5-5.5 oz-eq.	5.5-6.5 oz-eq.	6.5-7 oz-eq.	7-7.5 oz-eq.	7-7.5 oz-eq.	7.5-8 oz-eq.
Milk	2-3 c.	3 c.	3 c.	3 c.	3 c.	3 c.	3 c.	3 c.
Healthy Oils	4 tsp.	5 tsp.	5 tsp.	6 tsp.	6 tsp.	7 tsp.	8 tsp.	8 tsp.

Day/Date:

Breakfast: _____ Lunch: _____

Dinner: _____ Snack: _____

Group	Fruits	Vegetables	Grains	Meat & Beans	Milk	Oils
Goal Amount						
Estimate Your Total						
Increase ⇧ or Decrease? ⇩						

Physical Activity: _____ Spiritual Activity: _____

Steps/Miles/Minutes: _____

Day/Date:

Breakfast: _____ Lunch: _____

Dinner: _____ Snack: _____

Group	Fruits	Vegetables	Grains	Meat & Beans	Milk	Oils
Goal Amount						
Estimate Your Total						
Increase ⇧ or Decrease? ⇩						

Physical Activity: _____ Spiritual Activity: _____

Steps/Miles/Minutes: _____

Day/Date:

Breakfast: _____ Lunch: _____

Dinner: _____ Snack: _____

Group	Fruits	Vegetables	Grains	Meat & Beans	Milk	Oils
Goal Amount						
Estimate Your Total						
Increase ⇧ or Decrease? ⇩						

Physical Activity: _____ Spiritual Activity: _____

Steps/Miles/Minutes: _____

Day/Date: ___

Breakfast: _____

Lunch: _____

Dinner: _____

Snack: _____

Group	Fruits	Vegetables	Grains	Meat & Beans	Milk	Oils
Goal Amount						
Estimate Your Total						
Increase ⇧ or Decrease? ⇩						

Physical Activity: _____

Spiritual Activity: _____

Steps/Miles/Minutes: _____

Day/Date: ___

Breakfast: _____

Lunch: _____

Dinner: _____

Snack: _____

Group	Fruits	Vegetables	Grains	Meat & Beans	Milk	Oils
Goal Amount						
Estimate Your Total						
Increase ⇧ or Decrease? ⇩						

Physical Activity: _____

Spiritual Activity: _____

Steps/Miles/Minutes: _____

Day/Date: ___

Breakfast: _____

Lunch: _____

Dinner: _____

Snack: _____

Group	Fruits	Vegetables	Grains	Meat & Beans	Milk	Oils
Goal Amount						
Estimate Your Total						
Increase ⇧ or Decrease? ⇩						

Physical Activity: _____

Spiritual Activity: _____

Steps/Miles/Minutes: _____

Day/Date: ___

Breakfast: _____

Lunch: _____

Dinner: _____

Snack: _____

Group	Fruits	Vegetables	Grains	Meat & Beans	Milk	Oils
Goal Amount						
Estimate Your Total						
Increase ⇧ or Decrease? ⇩						

Physical Activity: _____

Spiritual Activity: _____

Steps/Miles/Minutes: _____

let's count our miles!

Join the 100-Mile Club this Session

Can't walk that mile yet? Don't be discouraged! There are exercises you can do to strengthen your body and burn those extra calories. Keep a record on your Live It Tracker of the number of minutes you do these common physical activities, convert those minutes to miles following the chart below, and then mark off each mile you have completed on the chart found on the back of the front cover. Report your miles to your 100-Mile Club representative when you first arrive each week. Remember, you are not competing with anyone else . . . just yourself. Your job is to strive to reach 100 miles before the last meeting in this session. You can do it—just keep on moving!

Walking

slowly, 2 mph	30 min. = 156 cal. = 1 mile
moderately, 3 mph	20 min. = 156 cal. = 1 mile
very briskly, 4 mph	15 min. = 156 cal. = 1 mile
speed walking	10 min. = 156 cal. = 1 mile
up stairs	13 min. = 159 cal. = 1 mile

Running/Jogging
10 min. = 156 cal. = 1 mile

Cycling Outdoors

slowly, <10 mph	20 min. = 156 cal. = 1 mile
light effort, 10-12 mph	12 min. = 156 cal. = 1 mile
moderate effort, 12-14 mph.	10 min. = 156 cal. = 1 mile
vigorous effort, 14-16 mph	7.5 min. = 156 cal. = 1 mile
very fast, 16-19 mph	6.5 min. = 152 cal. = 1 mile

Sports Activities

Playing tennis (singles)	10 min. = 156 cal. = 1 mile
Swimming	
light to moderate effort	11 min. = 152 cal. = 1 mile
fast, vigorous effort	7.5 min. = 156 cal. = 1 mile
Softball	15 min. = 156 cal. = 1 mile
Golf	20 min. = 156 cal = 1 mile
Rollerblading	6.5 min. = 152 cal. = 1 mile
Ice skating	11 min. = 152 cal. = 1 mile

Jumping rope	7.5 min. = 156 cal. = 1 mile
Basketball	12 min. = 156 cal. = 1 mile
Soccer (casual)	15 min. = 159 cal. = 1 mile

Around the House

Mowing grass	22 min. = 156 cal. = 1 mile
Mopping, sweeping, vacuuming	19.5 min. = 155 cal. = 1 mile
Cooking	40 min. =160 cal. = 1 mile
Gardening	19 min. = 156 cal. = 1 mile
Housework (general)	35 min. = 156 cal. = 1 mile
Ironing	45 min. = 153 cal. = 1 mile
Raking leaves	25 min. = 150 cal. = 1 mile
Washing car	23 min. = 156 cal. = 1 mile
Washing dishes	45 min. = 153 cal. = 1 mile

At the Gym

Stair machine	8.5 min. = 155 cal. = 1 mile
Stationary bike	
slowly, 10 mph	30 min. = 156 cal. = 1 mile
moderately, 10-13 mph	15 min. = 156 cal. = 1 mile
vigorously, 13-16 mph	7.5 min. = 156 cal. = 1 mile
briskly, 16-19 mph	6.5 min. = 156 cal. = 1 mile
Elliptical trainer	12 min. = 156 cal. = 1 mile
Weight machines (used vigorously)	13 min. = 152 cal.=1 mile
Aerobics	
low impact	15 min. = 156 cal. = 1 mile
high impact	12 min. = 156 cal. = 1 mile
water	20 min. = 156 cal. = 1 mile
Pilates	15 min. = 156 cal. = 1 mile
Raquetball (casual)	15 min. = 159 cal. = 1 mile
Stretching exercises	25 min. = 150 cal. = 1 mile
Weight lifting (also works for weight machines used moderately or gently)	30 min. = 156 cal. = 1 mile

Family Leisure

Playing piano	37 min. = 155 cal. = 1 mile
Jumping rope	10 min. = 152 cal. = 1 mile
Skating (moderate)	20 min. = 152 cal. = 1 mile
Swimming	
moderate	17 min. = 156 cal. = 1 mile
vigorous	10 min. = 148 cal. = 1 mile
Table tennis	25 min. = 150 cal. = 1 mile
Walk/run/play with kids	25 min. = 150 cal. = 1 mile